Pharmaceutical Drugs & Drug Therapy
for
Alternative Health Practitioners

**William A. Courson,
D.Ayur., DA (NAMA)**

Copyright © 2024 William Courson. All rights reserved.

The content of this book may not be reproduced, transmitted or duplicated in whole or in part without express written consent from the author or the publisher.

Under no circumstances will any blame or legal responsibility be maintained against the publisher, author or distributor of this book for any damages, injury, loss or reparation due to the use of information contained within, either directly or indirectly.

Legal Notice: This book is copyright protected. It is sold only for personal use. The user cannot amend, distribute, sell, use, quote or paraphrase any part of the content of this book without the express written permission of the author or publisher.

Disclaimer Notice: Please note that the information contained within this document is for educational and informational purposes only. All effort has been expended to present accurate, up-to-date, reliable and complete information. No warranties of any kind are declared or implied. Readers acknowledge that the author is not engaged in the rendering of professional advice. The content of this book has been derived from various sources. Please consult a licensed professional before utilizing any of the information contained in this book. By reading this document the reader agrees that under no circumstances is the author responsible for any losses, direct or indirect that are incurred because of the use of information contained within this document including, but not limited to, errors, omissions or inaccuracies.

ISBN No. 979-8336339970

CONTENTS

Introduction   13

Chapter 1: Introduction to Pharmaceutical Drugs   17
Understanding Pharmaceutical Drugs
History of Pharmaceutical Drugs
Importance of Pharmaceutical Drugs in Alternative Health Practices

Chapter 2: Drug Therapy Fundamentals   20
Principles of Drug Therapy
Drug Interactions and Side Effects
Dosage and Administration Guidelines

Chapter 3: Commonly Used Drugs   27
    Analgesics
    Acetaminophen
    Ibuprofen
    Naproxen
    Aspirin
    Opiates
    Other Analgesics

Antibiotics   42
    Penicillins
    Cephalosporins
    Macrolides
    Fluoroquinolones
    Sulfonamides
    Tetracyclines
    Other Antibiotics

Antivirals   49
    Categories of Antivirals Based on Action
    Categories of Antivirals Based on Virus Type

Antifungals   55
    Azoles
    Echinocandins
    Polyenes
    Allylamines
    Other Classes

Anti-Parasitical Drugs   58
    Antiprotozoal Agents
    Anthelmintic Agents
    Ant-Ectoparasitic Agents

Antidepressants and Anxiolytics   62
    Selective Serotonin Reuptake Inhibitors
    Selective Norepinephrine Reuptake Inhibitors
    Monoamine Oxidase Inhibitors
    Tricyclic Antidepressants
    Anxiolytics

Antipsychotics   67
    Typical Antipsychotics
    Atypical Antipsychotics
    Mood Stabilizers
    Stimulants

Cardiac Drugs   72
    Anti-Coagulants
    Anti-Platelet Agents
    ACE Inhibitors
    ARB Inhibitors
    ARN Inhibitors
    Beta Blockers
    Calcium Channel Blockers
    Statins
    Digitalis Preparations
    Diuretics
    Vasodilators

Respiratory Agents   80

    Bronchodilators
    Racemic Epinephrine
    Corticosteroids
    Mucolytics
    Cough Suppressants & Expectorants

Endocrine & Anti-Diabetic Drugs   87
    Anabolic Steroids
    Androgens
    Anti-Androgens
    Anti-Diabetic Drugs
    Calcitropic Hormones
    Estrogen
    Progesterone
    Obesity Drugs
    Thyroid Agents

Immunologic Drugs   100
    Immunostimulants
    Immunosuppressants

Neurological Drugs   108
    Cholinomimetics/cholinesterase antagonists
    Anticholinergics
    Adrenoreceptor agonists/sympathomimetics
    Adrenoreceptor antagonists
    Anti-Seizure Medications
    Alzheimers Drugs

Gastrointestinal Drugs   118
    Anti-Diarrheal
    Promotility Agents
    Digestive Enzymes
    Functional Bowel Disorder Agents
    Gallstone Solubilizing Agents
    5 Amino-Salicylates

Anti-Inflammatories   127
    Non-Steroidal Anti-Inflammatory Drugs (NSAIDs)

    Corticosteroids
    Disease Modifying Anti-Rheumatic Drugs
Antihistamines   131
    First Generation Anti-Histamines
    Second Generation Anti-Histamines
    Third Generation Anti-Histamines
    H2 Receptor Antagonists (H2 Blockers)
    Intranasal Anti-Histamines
    Ophthalmic Anti-Histamines
Anti-Neoplastic Drugs: Chemotherapy   135
    Alkylating Agents
    Anti-Metabolites
    Anti-Tumor Antibiotics
    Topoisomerase Inhibitors
    Mytotic Inhibitors
    Corticosteroids
    Miscellaneous Anti-Neoplastic Agents
    Targeted Therapies
    Hormone Therapy
    Immunotherapy
Topical Medications   139
    Skin Medications
    Ophthalmic Medications
    Otic (Ear) Medications
    Nasal Medications
    Oral Medications
    Vaginal Medications
    Rectal Medications
    Topical Neuro-Muscular Medications
    Topical Medications for Tobacco Cessation
Reproductive Management Drugs   145
Birth Control Drugs – Female
    Hormonal Methods
    Non-Hormonal Methods

    Herb-Drug Interactions
Birth Control Drugs – Male
    Hormonal Methods
    Non-Hormonal Methods
    Other Methods
Cancer Treatment Medicines   **149**
    Chemotherapy
    Targeted Therapies
    Hormone Therapies
    Immunotherapy
    Other Classes and Novel Approaches
    Cancer Drug-Herb Interactions
Prescription Vitamins and Minerals   **159**

Chapter 4: Herb-Drug Interactions   **162**

Chapter 5: Integrating Pharmaceutical Remedies   **260**
Monitoring and Evaluating Drug Therapy

Chapter 6: Herbal & Nutritional Supplements   **263**
Incorporating Nutritional Supplements
Combining Pharmaceuticals with Natural Therapies
Integrating Drug Therapy in Alternative Health Practice

Chapter 7: Resources and Further Reading   **270**

Bibliography
Glossary of Drug Terms

INTRODUCTION

In the evolving landscape of healthcare, alternative health practitioners are increasingly finding themselves at the crossroads of traditional healing practices and modern biomedical therapies. As more individuals seek holistic approaches to health, it becomes imperative for practitioners of alternative medicine to be well-versed not only in their own modalities but also in the pharmacological agents that dominate contemporary medical practice. This knowledge is essential for ensuring safe, effective, and integrative patient care.

Pharmaceutical Drugs and Drug Therapy for Alternative Health Practitioners aims to bridge this crucial knowledge gap. This book is designed to provide alternative health practitioners with a summary understanding of the pharmaceutical drugs that are commonly used in Western medicine. By familiarizing themselves with these medications, practitioners can better navigate the complex interactions between various conventional and alternative treatments, ultimately enhancing patient outcomes.

The realm of pharmaceutical drugs is vast and diverse, encompassing a wide range of medications that serve various therapeutic purposes. This book categorizes these drugs into two primary segments: prescription medications and over-the-counter (OTC) drugs.

Prescription medications are those drugs that require a healthcare provider's authorization for use. These include:

Analgesics
Antibiotics

Antivirals
Antifungals
Antiparasiticals
Antidepressants and Anxiolytics
Antipsychotics
Cardiac Drugs, Statins and Anti-Hypertensives
Respiratory Agents
Endocrine & Anti-Diabetic Drugs
Immunologic Drugs
Neurological Drugs
Gastrointestinal Drugs
Anti-Inflammatories
Antihistamines
Topical Medications
Chemotherapeutic agents
Prescription Vitamins and Minerals

Over-the-counter medications, on the other hand, are available without a prescription and are used to treat a wide range of minor ailments and symptoms. These include:

Analgesics: Such as acetaminophen and ibuprofen for pain relief.
Antihistamines: For allergy relief.
Decongestants: Used in treating nasal congestion.
Antacids and acid reducers: For managing heartburn and indigestion.
Laxatives: To relieve constipation.
Cough suppressants and expectorants: For managing cough and chest congestion.
Topical treatments: Including creams and ointments for skin conditions.

Each category of drug will be explored in detail, providing insights into their mechanisms of action, therapeutic uses, potential side effects, and interactions with other medications, including herbal remedies and supplements. By understanding these aspects, alternative health practitioners can make informed decisions and provide holistic care that respects and incorporates the benefits of both conventional and alternative therapies.

As the lines between different healthcare disciplines continue to blur, the need for collaborative and integrative approaches to patient care becomes ever more apparent. *Pharmaceutical Drugs and Drug Therapy for Alternative Health Practitioners* serves as an essential resource for those dedicated to embracing a comprehensive and informed approach to health and healing.

This book will hopefully equip non-medical practitioners with the knowledge and confidence to navigate the complexities of modern pharmacology, ultimately fostering a more harmonious and effective healthcare environment for all.

William Courson, D. Ayur., AD(NAMA)
Montclair, New Jersey USA
August 17, 2024

Chapter 1:
INTRODUCTION TO PHARMACEUTICAL DRUGS

Understanding Pharmaceutical Drugs

Pharmaceutical drugs are an essential component of modern healthcare, providing health care practitioners with effective tools to treat a wide range of health conditions. These drugs are designed to target specific symptoms or underlying causes of illness, helping to alleviate discomfort and improve overall well-being. It is important for alternative health practitioners to have a thorough understanding of pharmaceutical drugs, including their mechanisms of action, potential side effects, and appropriate dosages for different patient populations.

One of the key considerations when working with pharmaceutical drugs is understanding how they interact with the body. Drugs can exert their effects through a variety of mechanisms, such as targeting specific receptors in the body, inhibiting certain enzymes, or altering the production of key molecules.

By understanding these mechanisms, alternative health practitioners can better predict how a drug will affect a patient and tailor treatment plans accordingly.

In addition to understanding how pharmaceutical drugs work, alternative health practitioners must also be aware of potential side effects and contraindications. All drugs have the potential to cause adverse reactions in some individuals, ranging from mild to severe. By carefully monitoring patients for signs of side effects and adjusting treatment plans as needed, alternative health practitioners can minimize the risk of harm and maximize the benefits of pharmaceutical therapy.

Dosage is another important consideration when working with pharmaceutical drugs. Different patients may require different dosages of a drug based on factors such as age, weight, and overall health status. Alternative health practitioners should be aware of appropriate drug dosages to ensure that patients are receiving the optimal level of medication for their individual needs. Failure to do so can result in ineffective treatment or potential harm to the patient.

Pharmaceutical drugs are valuable tools for both conventiona and alternative health practitioners, offering effective treatment options for a wide range of health conditions. By understanding how these drugs work, monitoring for potential side effects, and being aware of dosages, alternative health practitioners can help to provide safe and effective care to their patients. It is essential for practitioners to stay informed about the developments in drug therapy and to approach drug therapy with a cautious and informed mindset.

History of Pharmaceutical Drugs

The history of pharmaceutical drugs dates back thousands of years to ancient civilizations such as the Egyptians, Greeks, and Chinese. These cultures were the first to recognize the healing properties of certain plants and minerals, laying the foundation for modern pharmaceutical medicine. The Egyptians, for example, used a variety of plant-based remedies to treat ailments ranging from headaches to infections. The Greeks, on the other hand, were known for their use of opium and other natural substances for pain relief.

During the Middle Ages, the practice of pharmacy began to take shape with the establishment of apothecaries and pharmacies. These early pharmacists would compound and dispense medications based on recipes passed down through generations. The Renaissance period saw advancements in pharmaceutical knowledge, with the discovery of new plants and minerals with medicinal properties. This era also saw the rise of the first pharmacopoeias, which standardized the preparation and dosing of pharmaceutical drugs.

The 19th century marked a turning point in the history of pharmaceutical drugs with the development of synthetic chemicals such as aspirin and morphine. These breakthroughs paved the way for the mass production of pharmaceuticals and the establishment of pharmaceutical companies. The 20th century brought further advancements in drug therapy with the discovery of antibiotics, vaccines, and other life-saving medications.

Today, pharmaceutical drugs have become an essential part of modern healthcare, providing effective treatments for a wide range of illnesses and conditions. Alternative health practitioners can benefit from incorporating pharmaceutical remedies into their practice, alongside other holistic therapies. By understanding the history of pharmaceutical drugs and how they have evolved over time, practitioners can make informed decisions about the best course of treatment for their patients.

The history of pharmaceutical drugs is a rich tapestry of ancient wisdom, scientific discovery, and medical innovation. Alternative health practitioners can draw upon this history to enhance their understanding of pharmaceutical remedies and their potential benefits for patients. By staying informed about the latest developments in drug therapy, practitioners can provide the best possible care for those seeking alternative health solutions.

Importance of Pharmaceutical Drugs in Alternative Health Practices

Pharmaceutical drugs play a crucial role in patient care, and provide practitioners with powerful tools to treat a wide range of health issues. While some may view pharmaceutical drugs as contradicting the principles of natural healing, they can actually complement alternative therapies and enhance patient outcomes. In many cases, pharmaceutical drugs are necessary to manage symptoms, alleviate pain, and improve overall well-being. By incorporating an awareness of pharmaceutical drugs into their practices, alternative health practitioners can offer comprehensive care that addresses both the root cause of a health issue and its symptoms.

One of the key benefits of pharmaceutical drugs is their ability to provide targeted and effective treatment. While natural remedies can be beneficial for certain conditions, pharmaceutical drugs offer a level of precision, potency and speed of action that is unmatched. For example, antibiotics can quickly and effectively treat bacterial infections, while pain medications can provide relief for acute or chronic pain. By becoming aware of of pharmaceutical drugs, alternative health practitioners can tailor treatment plans to meet the specific needs of each patient, leading to faster and more sustainable results.

Another important aspect of pharmaceutical drugs in alternative health practices is their ability to support and enhance the body's natural healing processes. While natural therapies such as acupuncture, massage, and herbal medicine can promote healing, pharmaceutical drugs can help to speed up the recovery process and minimize discomfort. For example, anti-inflammatory drugs can reduce swelling and pain, allowing the body to heal more quickly. By combining pharmaceutical drugs with holistic therapies, alternative health practitioners can create comprehensive treatment plans that address all aspects of a patient's health and well-being.

In addition to their therapeutic benefits, pharmaceutical drugs can also play a preventative role in alternative health practices. Many pharmaceutical drugs are used to manage chronic conditions such as diabetes, hypertension, and asthma, helping patients to maintain optimal health and prevent complications. By being aware of medications that address underlying health issues, alternative health practitioners can help patients to prevent future health problems and improve their quality of life. By incorporating an awareness of pharmaceutical drugs into their practices, alternative health practitioners can take a proactive approach to health and wellness, helping patients to stay healthy and vibrant for years to come.

Overall, pharmaceutical drugs are a valuable tools, offering a wide range of benefits that can enhance patient care and outcomes. By understanding the role that pharmaceutical drugs play in health care, practitioners can create more effective treatment plans that address both the symptoms and underlying causes of health issues. By integrating pharmaceutical drugs with natural therapies, practitioners can offer comprehensive care that supports the body's natural healing processes and promotes optimal health and well-being. With the right knowledge and approach, pharmaceutical drugs can be a powerful ally in the practice of alternative health.

Chapter 2:
DRUG THERAPY FUNDAMENTALS

Principles of Drug Therapy

In the world of alternative health practices, the use of pharmaceutical drugs is often a topic of debate. However, when used appropriately and in conjunction with other holistic therapies, pharmaceutical drugs can be a valuable tool in treating various health conditions. In this subchapter, we will discuss the principles of drug therapy for alternative health practitioners, providing a comprehensive guide on how to safely and effectively incorporate pharmaceutical remedies into your practice.

One of the key principles of drug therapy is understanding the mechanism of action of the pharmaceutical drug being used. Alternative health practitioners must have a thorough understanding of how a drug works in the body in order to properly assess its efficacy and potential side effects. This knowledge will also allow practitioners to make informed decisions about which drugs to prescribe based on their patients' individual needs and health conditions.

Another important principle of drug therapy is proper dosing and administration. Alternative health practitioners must be well-versed in the recommended dosage guidelines for each pharmaceutical drug they prescribe, as well as any potential interactions with other medications or supplements their patients may be taking. It is crucial to follow dosing instructions carefully to ensure the drug is effective and safe for the patient.

Monitoring and assessing the effectiveness of drug therapy is also essential for alternative health practitioners. Regular follow-up appointments and evaluations are necessary to track the progress of the patient's treatment and make any necessary adjustments to the drug regimen. This allows practitioners to ensure that the drug therapy is achieving the desired outcomes and address any potential issues or side effects that may arise.

Lastly, alternative health practitioners must always prioritize the well-being and safety of their patients when prescribing pharmaceutical drugs. This means being transparent about the potential risks and benefits of drug therapy, discussing alternative treatment options, and involving patients in the decision-making process. By adhering to these principles of drug therapy, alternative health practitioners can effectively integrate pharmaceutical remedies into their practice while maintaining a holistic approach to health and wellness.

Drug Interactions and Side Effects

Drug interactions and side effects are important considerations for alternative health practitioners when recommending pharmaceutical remedies to their patients. Understanding how different medications can interact with each other is crucial in order to avoid potentially harmful outcomes for patients.

It is essential for alternative health practitioners to be aware of potential drug interactions that can occur when multiple medications are taken together. Some drugs can have a synergistic effect when combined, leading to increased potency or side effects. On the other hand, certain medications may interact negatively with each other, diminishing the effectiveness of one or both drugs.

In addition to drug interactions, alternative health practitioners must also be knowledgeable about the potential side effects of pharmaceutical remedies. Every medication has the potential to cause side effects, ranging from mild to severe. It is important for practitioners to educate their patients about these potential side effects and monitor them closely for any adverse reactions.

Common side effects of pharmaceutical drugs can include nausea, dizziness, drowsiness, and allergic reactions. More serious side effects may include liver damage, kidney failure, or heart problems. Alternative health practitioners should be prepared to address any side effects that arise and work with patients to find alternative medications or treatment options if necessary.

By staying informed about drug interactions and side effects, alternative health practitioners can ensure the safety and well-being of their patients. It is crucial to always consult with a healthcare professional or pharmacist before recommending any pharmaceutical remedies to avoid potential complications. Patient safety should always be the top priority when considering drug therapy for alternative health practices.

Dosage and Administration Guidelines

Dosage and administration guidelines are crucial aspects of utilizing pharmaceutical remedies effectively in alternative health practices. It is essential for alternative health practitioners to understand the proper dosages and administration methods to ensure the safety and efficacy of drug therapy for their patients. In this subchapter, we will outline key considerations and recommendations for dosing and administering pharmaceutical drugs in alternative health settings.

When determining the appropriate dosage for a pharmaceutical remedy, alternative health practitioners must consider various factors such as the patient's age, weight, medical history, and the severity of the condition being treated. It is important to start with the lowest effective dose and titrate up as needed to achieve the desired therapeutic effect. Additionally, practitioners should be aware of any potential drug interactions or contraindications that may affect the dosage of the medication.

Administration guidelines for pharmaceutical remedies in alternative health practices involve the route of administration, frequency of dosing, and any specific instructions for taking the medication. Practitioners should educate their patients on how to properly administer the medication, whether it be orally, topically, intravenously, or through another route. Patients should also be informed of the importance of adhering to the prescribed dosing schedule to maximize the benefits of the treatment and minimize the risk of adverse effects.

Monitoring and adjusting the dosage of pharmaceutical remedies is an ongoing process that requires close observation and communication between the alternative health practitioner and the patient. Regular follow-up appointments should be scheduled to assess the patient's response to the medication, monitor for any side effects or adverse reactions, and make any necessary adjustments to the dosage or treatment plan. Alternative health practitioners should be prepared to modify the dosage or switch to a different medication if the initial treatment is not yielding the desired results.

In conclusion, dosage and administration guidelines play a critical role in the safe and effective use of pharmaceutical remedies in alternative health practices. Alternative health practitioners must be knowledgeable about dosing considerations, administration methods, and monitoring protocols to ensure the best possible outcomes for their patients. By following these guidelines and maintaining open communication with patients, alternative health practitioners can optimize the benefits of drug therapy while minimizing the risks associated with pharmaceutical remedies.

Chapter 3:
COMMONLY USED PHARMACEUTICAL REMEDIES

ANALGESICS

Pain management drugs are an essential tool for alternative health practitioners when it comes to treating patients with various conditions that cause discomfort and distress. These pharmaceutical remedies can help alleviate pain, improve quality of life, and promote healing in individuals seeking alternative approaches to healthcare. However, it is crucial for practitioners to have a thorough understanding of the different types of pain management drugs available, their mechanisms of action, potential side effects, and appropriate dosages for optimal patient outcomes.

Nonsteroidal anti-inflammatory drugs (NSAIDs) are commonly used in alternative medicine for their analgesic and anti-inflammatory properties. Examples of NSAIDs include ibuprofen, naproxen, and aspirin. These drugs work by inhibiting the production of prostaglandins, which are chemicals in the body that promote inflammation and pain. While NSAIDs can be effective for managing mild to moderate pain, practitioners should be cautious of potential side effects such as gastrointestinal ulcers, kidney damage, and cardiovascular risks, especially with long-term use.

Opioids are another class of pain management drugs that are commonly prescribed for severe pain, such as post-surgical discomfort or chronic conditions like cancer-

related pain. Examples of opioids include morphine, oxycodone, and fentanyl. These drugs work by binding to opioid receptors in the brain and spinal cord, effectively blocking pain signals and providing relief.
However, opioids come with a high risk of dependence, tolerance, and addiction, so practitioners should exercise caution when prescribing these medications and closely monitor patients for signs of misuse or abuse.

Muscle relaxants are another type of pain management drug that can be beneficial for patients experiencing muscle spasms, cramps, or tension-related pain. Examples of muscle relaxants include cyclobenzaprine, baclofen, and tizanidine. These drugs work by targeting the central nervous system to reduce muscle contractions and promote relaxation. While muscle relaxants can be effective for short-term relief of acute muscle pain, practitioners should be mindful of potential side effects such as drowsiness, dizziness, and impaired coordination, which can impact a patient's ability to perform daily activities.

Pain management drugs play a crucial role in the treatment of patients seeking alternative healthcare options for pain relief. Alternative health practitioners should be knowledgeable about the different types of pain management drugs available, their mechanisms of action, potential side effects, and appropriate dosages to ensure safe and effective treatment for their patients. By understanding the benefits and risks of various pharmaceutical remedies, practitioners can help alleviate pain, improve quality of life, and promote healing in individuals seeking alternative approaches to healthcare.

Major classifications of Analgesics include Non-Opioid & NSAIDs, Compounds, and Opioids

An analgesic or painkiller is any member of the group of drugs used to achieve analgesia, relief from pain. They are distinct from anesthetics, which temporarily affect, and in some instances completely eliminate, sensation.

Analgesic choice is also determined by the type of pain: For neuropathic pain, traditional analgesics are less effective, and there is often benefit from classes of drugs that and there is often benefit from classes of drugs that are not normally considered analgesics, such as tricyclic antidepressants and anticonvulsants.

Acetaminophen

Non-opioid analgesics include Acetaminophen (also known as Paracetamol, Tylenol), a medication used to mild to moderate pain. In combination with opioid pain medication, acetaminophen is now used for more severe pain such as cancer and post-surgical pain. It is typically used either by mouth or rectally but is also available intravenously. Effects last between two and four hours.

Acetaminophen is classified as a mild analgesic and is generally safe at recommended doses. Common side effects of acetaminophen are nausea and abdominal pain. Chronic consumption may result in a drop in hemoglobin level indicating possible gastrointestinal bleeding and abnormal liver function tests.

There is a consistent association of increased mortality as well as cardiovascular (stroke, myocardial infarction), gastrointestinal (ulcers, bleeding) and renal adverse effects with taking higher dose of Acetminophen. The drug may also increase the risk of developing hypertension.High doses may lead to toxicity, including liver failure. Paracetamol poisoning is the foremost cause of acute liver failure and accounts for most drug overdoses in the United States..

The recommended maximum daily dose for an adult is three to four gms.There is evidence of increased liver toxicity in acetaminophen overdose for phenobarbital, primidone, and possibly St John's wort and the anti-tubercular drug isoniazid. IT is widely sold under the brand names *Tylenol, Paracetamol, Calpol* and *Panado.*

Ibuprofen

Ibuprofen is a nonsteroidal anti-inflammatory drug (NSAID). It works by reducing hormones that cause inflammation and pain in the body. Ibuprofen is used to reduce fever and treat pain or inflammation caused by many conditions such as headache, toothache, back pain, arthritis, menstrual cramps, or minor injury. Ibuprofen should be avoided if one has ever had a severe allergic reaction after taking aspirin or an NSAID.

It should be used with caution in persons with heart disease, high blood pressure, high cholesterol, diabetes, or who are smokers of tobacco, are pregnant or breastfeeding (taking Ibuprofen during the last 20 weeks of pregnancy can evoke heart or kidney problems in the fetus and possible complications with pregnancy). It should be avoided by persons who have suffered a heart attack, stroke, or blood clot, who have stomach ulcers or bleeding, liver or kidney disease, asthma or by persons taking aspirin to prevent heart attack or stroke. Ibuprofen should not be given to a child under 6 months in age. Onset of effects is within an a half-hour and last for up to four hours

Common side effects with Ibuprofen include nausea, vomiting, and gas; or dizziness and headache. Infrequent but serious side effect include changes in vision, shortness of breath, swelling or rapid weight gain, skin rash, GI bleeding as indicated by bloody or tarry stools, coughing up blood or vomit that looks like coffee grounds; liver problems - nausea, upper stomach pain, itching, tired feeling, flu-like symptoms, loss of appetite, dark urine, clay-colored stools, jaundice (yellowing of the skin or eyes); anemia and kidney problems with little or no urinating, painful or difficult urination, swelling in the feet or ankles, and fatigue.

Interactions: Ibuprofen may interact negatively with Cyclosporine, *Cymbalta*, Lithium, Methotrexate, blood thinners (e.g., Warfarin, *Coumadin, Jantoven*); heart or blood pressure medication including a diuretic (e.g., HCTZ), steroid medications (e.g., fludrocortisone, prednisone), and *Zoloft*.

Ibuprofen is widely sold under the brand names *Motrin, Nuprin, Propinal* and *Advil*.

Naproxen

Naproxen is a nonsteroidal anti-inflammatory drug (NSAID) used to treat a variety of inflammatory conditions and symptoms that are due to excessive inflammation, such as pain and fever (naproxen has antipyretic properties) as well as migraine, osteoarthritis, kidney stones, rheumatoid arthritis, psoriatic arthritis, gout, ankylosing spondylitis, menstrual cramps, tendinitis, and bursitis. Naproxen sodium is used as a "bridge therapy" in medication-overuse headache to slowly take patients off other medications.

Naproxen is a nonselective COX inhibitor. It is in the propionic acid class of medications. As an NSAID, naproxen exerts its anti-inflammatory action by reducing the production of inflammatory mediators called prostaglandins. It is metabolized by the liver to inactive metabolites.

Naproxen should be avoided in people with kidney problems nor in the third trimester of pregnancy. Heavy use is associated with increased risk of end-stage renal disease and kidney failure. Naproxen may cause muscle cramps in the legs in 3% of people. As with other NSAIDs, naproxen can cause gastrointestinal problems, such as heartburn, constipation, diarrhea, ulcers and stomach bleeding.

Naproxen should be taken orally with food to decrease the risk of gastrointestinal side effects. Persons with a history of ulcers or inflammatory bowel disease should consult a doctor before taking naproxen. Naproxen poses an intermediate risk of stomach ulcers (compared with ibuprofen, which is low-risk) and to reduce the risk of ulceration, it is often combined with a proton-pump inhibitor.

Common side effects include dizziness, headache, bruising, allergic reactions, heartburn, and stomach pain. Severe side effects include an increased risk of heart disease, stroke, gastrointestinal bleeding. Rarely, anemia, shortness of breath and body rash are seen.

Naproxen may interact with antidepressants, Lithium, Methotrexate, Probenecid, Warfarin, Coumadin and other blood thinners, heart or blood pressure medications including diuretics (e.g., HCTZ), or steroid medicines (e.g., Prednisone, Fludrocortizone, etc.) as well as Cholestyramine, Cyclosporine, Digoxin, Pemetrexed, Phenytoin or similar seizure medications and Insulin or other oral diabetes medicine. NSAIDs such as naproxen may interfere with and reduce the efficacy of SSRI antidepressants, as well as increase the risk of bleeding greater than the individual bleeding risk of either class of agent when taken together.

Alcohol consumption increases the risk of gastrointestinal bleeding when combined with NSAIDs like naproxen in a dose-dependent manner (that is, the higher the dose of naproxen, the more likely to provoke a bleed.

Naproxen is widely sold under the brand names *Aleve, Anaprox, Naprelyn* and *Naprosyn.*

Aspirin

Aspirin, also known as acetylsalicylic acid (ASA), is a medication used to reduce pain, fever, or inflammation. Specific inflammatory conditions which aspirin is used to treat include Kawasaki disease, pericarditis, and rheumatic fever.

Aspirin is an effective analgesic for acute pain, although it is generally considered inferior to ibuprofen because aspirin is more likely to cause gastrointestinal bleeding. Aspirin is generally ineffective for those pains caused by muscle cramps, bloating, gastric distension, or acute skin irritation. Aspirin given shortly after a heart attack decreases the risk of death. Aspirin is also used long-term to help prevent further heart attacks, ischaemic strokes, and blood clots in people at high risk.

Aspirin works similarly to other NSAIDs but also suppresses the normal functioning of platelets. There is some evidence that has shown that aspirin as a chemoprotective agent may reduce overall cancer incidence and mortality in colorectal, esophageal and gastric cancers with smaller effects on prostate, breast and lung cancer.

The most common adverse effect is an upset stomach. More significant side effects include stomach ulcers, stomach bleeding, and worsening asthma. Bleeding risk is greater among those who are older, drink alcohol, take other NSAIDs, or are on other blood thinners. Aspirin is not recommended in the last part of pregnancy. It is not generally recommended in children with infections because of the risk of Reye's syndrome. High doses may result in ringing in the ears.

Opiates

The chief use of opiates is in the treatment of moderate to severe pain, and in some instances severe diarrhea and coughing. Opiates may be either natural, synthetic or semi-synthetic.

Natural Opiates include Opium derived from poppy seed plants, which contain a high concentration of morphine-derived alkaloids, which accounts for why morphine is one of the strongest opiates in existence. Codeine-derived alkaloids make up the second highest concentration. Technically speaking, only natural opiates quality as actual opiate drugs; however, any drug derived and/or synthesized to act as an opiate material falls within the opiate category. These natural products come from the alkaloid materials found in the opium poppy seed plant itself. Natural opiate drug types include:

Codeine
Morphine
Oripavine
Thebaine

Synthetic Opiate Drugs: The synthetic opiates list contains a wide assortment of manufactured drugs, each of which targets different intensities and types of pain symptoms. Though manufactured to resemble natural alkaloid substances, synthetic drug formulations can carry considerably higher potencies than natural alkaloids. Synthetic opiate drug types include:

Lortab
Demerol
Atarax
Dilaudid
Fentanyl

Synthetic opiates also include five of the most often prescribed opiate addiction treatment drugs: Methadone,

Suboxone, *Subutex*, Naltrexone, and Naloxone. Whereas methadone, Suboxone and *Subutex* act as substitutes for addictive opiates, naltrexone blocks opiates from stimulating cell receptor sites while naloxone expels existing opiate materials from cell sites.

Semisynthetic opiates contain small amounts of natural opium alkaloids combined with synthetic agents. Natural alkaloids used in the making of semisynthetic opiates include Codeine (for hydrocodone), Morphine (for hydromorphone) and Thebaine (for oxymorphone and oxycodone) The semisynthetic opiates list includes the following drugs:

Oxycodone (*Oxycontin, Percocet*)
Oxymorphone (*Opana*)
Hydromorphone (*Dilaudid, Exalgo*)
Hydrocodone (*Vicodin, Lortab*)
Tramadol (*Ultram, Ultracet*)

Nausea, vomiting, dizziness and sedation are among the most common reactions to the drugs, but a multitude of health consequences can accompany long-term opiate use, but many of the risks are seen more acutely. Even a first-time user can experience respiratory arrest, for example. Opioid painkillers can lead to respiratory depression, a slowing of breathing. At sufficient doses, respiratory arrest can result which can easily prove fatal, or result in debilitating organ system injury.

Opiates affect the muscles of the digestive system, leading to constipation due to a slowing of digestive transit. The slowed gastrointestinal motility and chronic constipation associated with opiate abuse can also place users at heightened risk for more serious conditions, such as small bowel obstruction, perforation and resultant peritonitis. Nausea also occurs frequently in many users of opioids, along with sudden, uncontrollable vomiting.

Paradoxically, the chronic use of opioids can lead to the development of hyperalgesia, a syndrome of increased sensitivity to pain. Opioid use is also associated with psychomotor impairment, an overall slowing of a person's physical movements and loss of coordination, and sedation with impaired motor reflexes.Opioid painkillers are known to be associated with suppression of the immune system, as opioid receptors are involved with regulation of immunity.

Because many opioid painkillers are combined with acetaminophen, excessive use of these drugs can cause liver damage from acetaminophen toxicity. Damage to the liver from acetaminophen toxicity is an undeniable risk of taking excessive doses of many prescription painkillers such as *Lortab*, *Norco* and *Vicodin*. The use of alcohol further decreases the liver's ability to process the toxic combination of ethanol and acetaminophen.

While many medications can interact with opioid medications, chief examples are:

Alcohol
Anti-seizure medications, such as carbamazepine, topiramate and lamotrigine (*Lamictal*)
Benzodazepines, such as diazepam (*Valium*), lorazepam (*Ativan*),(*Xanax*) and clonazepam (*Klonopin*)
Certain antibiotics, including clarithromycin
Certain antidepressants

Certain antifungals, including itraconazole, voriconazole and ketoconazole
Certain antiretroviral drugs used for HIV infection, including atazanavir (*Reyataz*), indinavir (*Crixivan*) and ritonavir (*Norvir*)
Drugs for sleeping problems, such as *Ambien, Edluar*, Lunesta and *Sonata*
Drugs used to treat psychiatric disorders, such as haloperidol (Haldol), clozapine (*Clozaril, Versacloz*), aripiprazole (*Abilify*) and quetiapine (*Seroquel*)
Medications used to treat certain types of nerve pain, such as gabapentin (*Neurontin, Gralise*) and pregabalin (*Lyrica*)
Muscle relaxers, such as cyclobenzaprine (*Amrix* and *Baclofen*)
Other opioid medications

Other Analgesics

Tramadol (*Ultram*) is a synthetic opiate agonist and inhibitor of norepinephrine and serotonin uptake; not an opium derivative or a semisynthetic derivative of morphine or thebaine. It for the management of pain that is severe enough to require an opiate analgesic and for which alternative treatment options (e.g., nonopiate analgesics) have not been, or are not expected to be, adequate or tolerated. Efficacy established in patients with moderately severe acute or chronic pain, including postoperative, gynecologic, obstetric, and cancer pain. There are numerous potential side effects, and misuse can have lethal results.

Gabapentin, sold under the brand name *Neurontin* among others, is actually an anticonvulsant medication primarily used to treat seizures and neuropathic pain. It is a first-line medication for the treatment of neuropathic pain caused by diabetic neuropathy, postherpetic neuralgia, and central pain (a neurological condition consisting of constant, moderate to severe pain due to damage to the central nervous system).It is moderately effective: about 30-40% of those given gabapentin have a meaningful benefit. It is often prescribed off-label for RLS, anxiety and bipolar disorder.

Diclofenac is an NSAID used to reduce inflammation and as an analgesic to reduce pain in conditions such as arthritis, acute injury, and other inflammatory conditions. It is available in several formulations, including oral and topical forms. Diclofenac works by inhibiting the enzyme cyclooxygenase (COX), which is involved in the synthesis of prostaglandins. Prostaglandins are mediators of inflammation, pain, and fever. By reducing their production, diclofenac helps to decrease inflammation and alleviate pain. It is used in such pathologies such as osteoarthritis, rheumatoid arthritis, ankylosing spondylitis, acute musculoskeletal pain, dysmenorrhea, post-operative pain and migraine. Long-term use or high doses can increase the risk of cardiovascular events (such as heart attack or stroke) and gastrointestinal bleeding or ulcers.

It is contraindicated in patients with known hypersensitivity to diclofenac or other NSAIDs, a history of gastrointestinal bleeding or ulcers, heart failure, kidney, or liver disease and should be used with caution in patients with cardiovascular risk factors. *Zipsor* and *Cataflam* are oral forms, and *Voltaren* and *Flector* are topical applications. *Arthrotec* is a combination of diclofenac and misoprostol (a synthetic prostaglandin used to protect the stomach lining), used to treat arthritis while reducing the risk of stomach ulcers.

Meloxicam is a nonsteroidal anti-inflammatory drug (NSAID) used to treat pain and inflammation associated with various forms of arthritis, such as osteoarthritis and rheumatoid arthritis. It is available in oral formulations (tablets and capsules) and as an injectable form. Meloxicam works by inhibiting the enzyme cyclooxygenase (COX), specifically COX-2 more selectively than COX-1. This inhibition reduces the production of prostaglandins, which are chemicals in the body that promote inflammation, pain, and fever. By reducing the levels of prostaglandins, meloxicam helps to decrease inflammation and alleviate pain.

The dosage of meloxicam depends on the specific condition being treated and the patient's overall health. It is typically taken once daily, with or without food. It is important to follow the prescribing healthcare provider's instructions and not to exceed the recommended dose. Meloxicam should be used under the guidance of a healthcare professional, who will consider the benefits and potential risks for each individual patient. Regular monitoring may be necessary for those on long-term treatment, especially for kidney and liver function, as well as cardiovascular health. It is commonly used in osteoarthritis, rheumatoid arthritis and juvenile idiopathic arthritis (in children). Common side effects of meloxicam include stomach pain, indigestion, nausea, diarrhea, constipation, headache, dizziness, upper respiratory tract infections, and rash. Serious side effects can include increased risk of cardiovascular events (such as heart attack or stroke) with long-term use or high doses, gastrointestinal bleeding or ulcers and kidney and liver damage. *Mobic*, *Vivlodex* and *Qmiiz* are widely available oral forms.

Ketamine is a medication that was originally developed as an anesthetic but is now used in various contexts. It is used in surgery and emergency medicine to induce and maintain anesthesia because it provides sedation, pain relief, and memory loss (amnesia) without significantly depressing breathing. In pain management it is sometimes given at low doses for severe or chronic pain, especially when other painkillers are not effective.

In recent years, ketamine (or its derivative esketamine) has been used "off-label" or in specialized clinics to treat severe treatment-resistant depression, PTSD, and suicidal thoughts. It's given in carefully controlled doses, either as an IV infusion or nasal spray (FDA-approved esketamine, brand name *Spravato*). Ketamine works mainly by blocking a brain receptor called NMDA (N-methyl-D-aspartate), which affects glutamate, a neurotransmitter that plays a role in pain and mood regulation.

Ketamine is sometimes misused as a recreational drug due to its dissociative and hallucinogenic effects: it can make its user feel detached from reality, have vivid dreams, or experience an "out-of-body" feeling. At higher doses, this can be dangerous and lead to what's called a "K-hole" (a deep dissociative state).

When used medically, ketamine is generally safe under supervision but can raise blood pressure and heart rate, and in repeated misuse, it may cause urinary tract and bladder issuess, cognitive changes, or dependence.

ANTIBIOTICS

Antibiotics and antivirals play a crucial role in modern medicine, including the practice of alternative health. These pharmaceutical drugs are essential in treating bacterial and viral infections, helping to alleviate symptoms and promote healing. Alternative health practitioners can benefit from understanding how these medications work and when they may be appropriate for their patients.

Antibiotics are medications that are used to treat bacterial infections by either killing the bacteria or preventing their growth. It is important for alternative health practitioners to be aware of when antibiotics are necessary and when they may not be the best course of treatment. Overuse of antibiotics can lead to antibiotic resistance, making these medications less effective in the long run. Practitioners should always consider the potential risks and benefits of antibiotic therapy and use them judiciously.

Correct use of antibiotics is absolutely essential to help reduce antibiotic resistance. Germs become resistant to antibiotics over time, which then makes them less effective, and the World Health Organization (WHO) says "the world urgently needs to change the way it prescribes and uses antibiotics" as antibiotic resistance is a major global threat.

The choice of antibiotic mainly depends on which infection and the microbe (bacterium or parasite) that is causing the infection, as each antibiotic is effective only against certain bacteria and parasites. For example, in cases of pneumonia, one must know what kinds of bacteria are causative. Other factors that influence the choice of an antibiotic include:

How severe the infection is
How well the patient's kidneys and liver are functioning
Dosing schedule
Other medications being taken
Common side-effects
A history of allergy to a certain type of antibiotic.
Pregnant or lactation
Pattern of infection in the community
Pattern of resistance to antibiotics by microbes in the area

The discovery by Alexander Fleming of the first true antibiotic—penicillin—in 1928 was one of the most life-changing events of the 20th century. Before its discovery, when bacterial infections attacked death was the rule rather than the exception. The first Penicillin gave rise to an entire class of antibiotics collectively known as penicillins. Penicillins are derived from a specific mold (a type of fungi)—*Penicillium*. They are widely useful antibiotics that are often a first choice for several types of infections. This includes skin, respiratory, ear, STDs and dental infections. They are highly effective against familiar organisms, such as staph and strep. Rashes and allergic reactions are common with penicillins. Other common side effects include diarrhea, nausea, and abdominal pain.

Penicillins

Penicillin does not combat all types microbes and is most effective against gram-positive bacteria. Penicillin kills

bacteria by disrupting the peptidoglycan cross-linking process. Gram negative bacteria, including E. (Escherichia) Coli, have thin polysaccharide walls overlaid by thin layers of lipopolysaccharides which make them resistant to Penicillin
Side effects may include diarrhea, nausea, heartburn, and abdominal pain.

Examples of Penicillins include:

Amoxicillin
Ampicillin
Penicillin G
Penicillin V
Penicillin VK

Cephalosporins

Cephalosporins are related to penicillins. Like penicillins, cephalosporins originally came from a fungus— *Cephalosporium*.

There are five generations of cephalosporins. Each generation covers different types of bacteria. As a result, the class can treat a variety of infections, from strep throat and skin infections to major infections like meningitis and encephalitis. Because they are related to penicillins, some people with penicillin allergies may also react to cephalosporins exhibiting side effects include diarrhea, nausea, heartburn, and abdominal pain. Examples of cephalosporins include:

Cefixime
Cefpodoxime

Cefuroxime
Cephalexin

Macrolides

Macrolides are a completely different class of antibiotics from the penicillins and cyclosporins. but they effectively treat many of the same infections. This includes respiratory, ear, skin, infections and STDs. Thus,, they are very useful for people with allergies to the foregoing antibiotics. They are also useful when bacteria develop resistance to the same antibiotics (eg, Vancomycin for MRSA). Common side effects include nausea, vomiting, stomach pain, and diarrhea, the last occasionally provoked by c. difficile overgrowth.

Macrolides have a large number of of drug interactions: over 590 documented to date. Potentially lethal ones include *Lipitor* (Atorvastatin), *Miralax* (Polyethelene Glycol), *Xanax* (Alprazolam) and *Zofran* (Ondansetron).

Azithromycin ('*Z-pak*')
Clarithromycin
Erythromycin
Vancomycin

Flouroquinolones

Fluoroquinolones—or quinolones—are active against a very wide variety of bacteria. This makes them useful for treating infections when other antibiotics have failed, and are also an alternative when patients present with allergies to other antibiotics. They can treat anything from eye infections to pneumonia to skin, sinus, joint, urinary or gynecologic infections and many more.

This class can be a problem for people with certain heart conditions and with some other medicines including omeprazole, *metformin, citalopram,* warfarin, *flagyl,* amiodorone, and tizanadine, among others.

Common side effects include stomach upset or pain, diarrhea, headache and drowsiness.
Examples of fluoroquinolones include:

Ciprofloxacin
Levofloxacin
Moxifloxacin

Sulfonamides

Derived from the chemical sulfanilamide, 'sulfa drugs' have been around about as long as penicillin. Technically, sulfonamides don't kill bacteria the way other antibiotics do. Instead of being antibiotic, , they are bacteriostatic—they stop bacterial growth and rely on the immune to disable invasive bacteria. They are very good topical treatments for burns and vaginal or eye infections. They can also treat UTIs (urinary tract infections) and traveler's diarrhea. However, resistance is common with this class.

Common side effects include diarrhea, nausea, rash, and sun sensitivity. Allergies are also common with the group.

Drug reactions include *Lisinopril, Metformin, Digosxin, Cyclosporin* and others.

Examples of sulfonamides include:

Sulfacetamide (*Ovase, Cetamide, Bleph-10*)
Sulfadiazine (*Silvadene, Thermazine*)
Sulfamethoxazole-Trimethoprim (*Bactrim*)

Tetracycline

These antibiotics come from a species of bacteria called *Streptomyces,* a bacterium that produces an antibiotic substance that kills other bacteria. Tetracyclines are bacteriostatic, like the sulfonamides.

They treat various infections, such as respiratory, skin and genital infections. They also treat unusual gram negative infections, including Lyme disease, malaria, anthrax, cholera, and plague.

They have noninfectious uses as well, such as treating rosacea. Common side effects include stomach pain or upset, sun sensitivity, and yeast infections.
Serious drug interactions exist with Strontium Ranelate, Retinoids and Live Typhoid Vaccine, among many others.

Examples of tetracyclines include:

Doxycycline
Minocycline
Tetracycline

Othe Antibiotics

Clindamycin *(Cliocin)*: Clindamycin is in a class of medications called lincomycin antibiotics. It works by slowing or stopping the growth of bacteria and is used to treat certain types of bacterial infections, including infections of the bones and joints, lungs, skin, blood, female reproductive organs (pelvic inflammatory disease), strep throat, endocarditis, and other internal organs as well as anthrax and malaria.It can treat some cases of methicillin-resistant Staphylococcus aureus (MRSA).

Metronidazole *(Flagyl)*: Metronidazole, marketed under the brand name Flagyl among others, is an antibiotic and antiprotozoal medication. It is used either alone or with other antibiotics to treat pelvic inflammatory disease, endocarditis, and bacterial vaginosis. It is effective for parasites: dracunculiasis, giardiasis, trichomoniasis, and amebiasis. It is an option for a first episode of mild-to-moderate Clostridium difficile. Common side effects include nausea, a metallic taste, loss of appetite, and headaches.Occasionally seizures or allergies to the medication may occur.

Nitrofurantoin *(Furadantin, Macrodantin)*: Current uses include the treatment of uncomplicated urinary tract infections (UTIs) and prophylaxis against UTIs in people prone to recurrent UTIs. Increasing bacterial antibiotic resistance to other commonly used agents, such as fluoroquinolones and trimethoprim/sulfamethoxazole, has led to increased interest in using nitrofurantoin. The efficacy of nitrofurantoin in treating UTIs combined with a low rate of bacterial resistance to this agent makes it one of the first-line agents for treating uncomplicated UTIs. It is a wide-sprectrum antibiotic, but is ineffective against Enterobacter, Proteus and Pseudomonas bacteria.

ANTIVIRALS

Antivirals are medications that are used to treat viral infections by inhibiting the replication of the virus. While antibiotics are ineffective against viruses, antivirals can be effective in treating certain viral infections such as influenza or herpes. Alternative health practitioners should be familiar with the different types of antiviral drugs available and their indications for use. It is important to note that antivirals are most effective when started early in the course of the infection.

Antivirals can protect one from getting viral infections or spreading a virus to others. These tiny (microscopic) infectious agents grow and multiply only inside living cells of an organism. Viruses have receptors that allow them to attach to healthy (host) cells in your body. Once a virus attaches to and enters a host cell, it can replicate (make copies of itself). The host cell dies, and the virus infects other healthy cells. Antiviral medicines work differently depending on the drug and virus type.

Antivirals can:

Block receptors so viruses can't bind to and enter healthy cells.
Boost the immune system, helping it fight off a viral infection.
Lower the viral load (amount of active virus) in the body.

Most viruses are self-resolving. Prescribed use antivirals to treat chronic or life-threatening viral infections, including:

Coronaviruses like COVID-19.
Ebola
Influenza, including H1N1 (swine flu).
Genital herpes.
Hepatitis B and hepatitis C.
Human immunodeficiency virus (HIV).

Antiviral drugs can ease symptoms and shorten the period of active illness with viral infections like Influenza and Ebola and can rid the body of these viruses. Viral infections like HIV, Hepatitis and Herpes are chronic. Antivirals cannot rid the body of the virus, which remains in your body; however, antivirals can render the virus latent (inactive) so that infected persons have few, if any, symptoms. Symptoms that develop while you take antivirals may be less severe or abate faster. Antiviral drugs can prevent certain viral infections after a suspected or known exposure.

Antvirals work in one of a variety of ways:

One anti-viral strategy is to interfere with the ability of a virus to infiltrate a target cell. Another is to target the processes that synthesize virus components after a virus invades a cell by developing nucleotide analogues that look like the building blocks of the virus RNA or DNA, but deactivate the enzymes that synthesize the RNA or DNA. The first successful antiviral, *Aciclovir*, is one of these.

Yet another antiviral technique is based on *ribozymes*, which are enzymes that will cut apart viral RNA or DNA at selected sites. In their natural course, ribozymes are used as part of the viral manufacturing sequence, but these synthetic ribozymes are designed to cut RNA and DNA at sites that will disable them.

Antivirals can be categorized based on their mechanism of action, and the types of viruses they target. Here are the main categories:

Categories of Antivirals Based on Mechanism of Action

Nucleoside/Nucleotide Analogues:
Mimic the building blocks of viral DNA or RNA, getting incorporated into the viral genome and causing premature termination of replication.
Examples: Acyclovir (herpesviruses), Zidovudine (HIV), Sofosbuvir (Hepatitis C)

Non-Nucleoside Reverse Transcriptase Inhibitors (NNRTIs):
Bind to and inhibit reverse transcriptase, an enzyme crucial for viral replication in retroviruses like HIV.
Examples: Efavirenz, Nevirapine

Protease Inhibitors:
Inhibit viral proteases, enzymes necessary for the maturation of infectious viral particles.
Examples: Ritonavir (HIV), Simeprevir (Hepatitis C)

Integrase Inhibitors:
Inhibit integrase, an enzyme that integrates viral DNA into the host genome.
Examples: Raltegravir, Dolutegravir (both for HIV)

Entry Inhibitors:

Block the virus from entering host cells.
Examples: Enfuvirtide (HIV), Maraviroc (HIV)

Fusion Inhibitors:
Prevent the fusion of the viral membrane with the host cell membrane.
Example: Enfuvirtide (HIV)

Neuraminidase Inhibitors:
Inhibit neuraminidase, an enzyme necessary for the release of new viral particles from infected cells.
Examples: Oseltamivir, Zanamivir (both for Influenza)

Uncoating Inhibitors:
Inhibit the uncoating process of the virus, preventing it from releasing its genetic material into the host cell.
Example: Amantadine (Influenza A)

Categories Based on Based on Target Virus Type

Anti-Herpesvirus Agents:
Examples: Acyclovir, Valacyclovir, Famciclovir

Anti-Retroviral Agents (HIV):
Examples: Zidovudine, Efavirenz, Ritonavir, Raltegravir

Anti-Influenza Agents:
Examples: Oseltamivir, Zanamivir, Amantadine

Anti-Hepatitis Agents:
Hepatitis B: Tenofovir, Entecavir
Hepatitis C: Sofosbuvir, Simeprevir, Ribavirin

Broad-Spectrum Antivirals:

Effective against multiple virus types.
Example: Ribavirin (used for RSV, Hepatitis C, some hemorrhagic fevers)

Antiviral drugs have a great many potential side effect of varying seriousness, which include:

Abdominal or stomach pain
Hallucinations
Black, tarry stools
Headaches
Blood in urine or stools
Hives
Chills
Fever
Sore throat
Increased thirst
Confusion
Joint or muscle pain
Cough
Loss of appetite
Convulsions (seizures)
Nausea or vomiting
Decreased frequency /amount of urine
Pinpoint red spots on skin
Diarrhea.
Skin rash.
Dizziness.
Trembling
Dry mouth
Unusual tiredness or weakness
Fatigue
Unusual bleeding or bruising

Antiviral drug development is now progressing at the pace antibiotics were 30 years ago. At present, there are some 60 antiviral drug preparations that have been approved by the US FDA, almost half of which are used for the treatment of HIV infections. The remaining half are used for the treatment of HBV (Hepatitis B), herpes simplex virus (HSV), varicella-zoster virus (VZV), cytomegalovirus (CMV), influenza and HCV (Hepatitis C) infections. These include (among others):

Abacavir *(Ziagen)* - HIV, VZV
Acyclovir *(Zovirax)* - Herpes infections
Baloxivir (*Xofluza*) - Influenza
Efavirenz *(Sustiva)* - HIV
Famciclovir *(Famvir)* - Herpes infections
Lopinivir (*Kaletra*) - HIV
Oseltamvir (*Tamiflu*) - Influenza
Peramivir (*Rapivab*) - Influenza
Remdesivir (*Veklury*) - Covid 19 & other viral infections)
Tenofovir (*Viread*) - HIV, HBV, HCV
Valacyclovir *(Valtrex)*   - Herpes infections, VZV
Vaganciclovir (*Valcyte*) - CMV

Zenamivir (*Relenza*) - Influenza

When prescribing antibiotics or antivirals, alternative health practitioners should consider the individual needs and circumstances of each patient. It is important to take into account factors such as allergies, drug interactions, and potential side effects when selecting a medication. Practitioners should also educate their patients on the proper use of these medications, including dosage instructions and potential side effects to watch for.

Antibiotics and antivirals are valuable tools in the treatment of bacterial and viral infections. Alternative health practitioners can benefit from understanding the role of these medications in modern medicine and how they can be used effectively and responsibly. By staying informed and making thoughtful decisions about when to use antibiotics and antivirals, practitioners can provide their patients with safe and effective care.

ANTIFUNGALS

Antifungals are a crucial class of pharmaceutical drugs that are used to treat fungal infections in the body. As Alternative Health Practitioners, it is important to have a thorough understanding of antifungals and their use in managing various fungal conditions. This subchapter will delve into the different types of antifungal medications available, their mechanisms of action, common side effects, and considerations for their use in alternative health practices.

There are several types of antifungal medications, each targeting different aspects of fungal growth and replication. Some common classes of antifungals include azoles, echinocandins, and polyenes.

Azoles

Azoles work by inhibiting the synthesis of ergosterol, a crucial component of fungal cell membranes, and are widely used to treat a variety of fungal infections, including those affecting the skin, nails, and mucous membranes. Commonly prescribed azole antifungals include:

Fluconazole (*Diflucan, Trican, Monicure*)
Itraconazole (*Sporanox, Onmel*)
Ketoconazole (*Nizoral, Extina, Xolegel*)
Voriconazole (*Vfend*)
Posaconazole (*Noxafil*)
Isavuconazole (*Cresemba*)
Clotrimazole (*Lotrimin, Mycelex, Canesten*)
Miconazole (*Monistat, Desenex, Micatin*)
Econazole (*Spectazole*)
Tioconazole (*Vagistat-1, Trosyd*)

Echinocandins

Echinocandins target the enzyme responsible for cell wall synthesis in fungi, while polyenes disrupt the cell membrane integrity, leading to cell death. Echinocandin antifungals are a newer class of antifungal medications that are primarily used to treat invasive fungal infections, particularly those caused by Candida and Aspergillus species. Commonly sold echonocandins include:

Caspofungin (*Cancidas*)
Micafungin (*Mycamine*)
Anidulafungin (*Eraxis*)

Polyenes

Polyene antifungals are a class of antifungal medications primarily used to treat serious fungal infections. These polyene antifungals are widely used to treat systemic fungal infections. Here are the most widely sold polyene antifungals and their brand names:

Amphotericin B (*Funngizone, Ambisome, Abelcet, Amphotec*)
Nystatin (*Mycostatin, Bio-Statin, Nystop*)
Natamycin (*Natacyn*)

Allylamines

Mechanism: Inhibit squalene epoxidase, interfering with ergosterol synthesis and disrupting cell membrane integrity. Examples: *Terbinafine, Naftifine*

Other Classes

Pyrimidine Analogues: Flucytosine (inhibits DNA and RNA synthesis)
Griseofulvin: Disrupts microtubule function, inhibiting fungal cell division.

By understanding the mechanisms of action of these different classes of antifungals, Alternative Health Practitioners can better tailor their treatment plans to individual patients.
When dealing with a client taking antifungal medications, it is important to consider potential side effects that may arise. Common side effects of antifungals include gastrointestinal upset, liver toxicity, and allergic reactions. Alternative Health Practitioners should monitor patients closely for any signs of adverse reactions and adjust treatment accordingly. Additionally, drug interactions with antifungals are common, so it is important to review

patients' medication histories before prescribing these drugs.

In alternative health practices, antifungals may be seen to be used to treat a wide range of fungal infections, including yeast infections, fungal nail infections, and systemic fungal infections. It is important for Alternative Health Practitioners to consider the underlying cause of the fungal infection and address any contributing factors to prevent recurrence. Antifungals may be used in conjunction with other natural therapies, such as probiotics and herbal remedies, to support the body's immune system and restore balance.

In conclusion, antifungal medications are an essential tool in the treatment of fungal infections for Alternative Health Practitioners. By understanding the different classes of antifungals, their mechanisms of action, common side effects, and considerations for use in alternative health practices, practitioners can provide effective and holistic care for patients with fungal infections. It is important to approach treatment with a comprehensive and individualized approach, taking into account the patient's overall health and wellness.

ANTI-PARASITICAL DRUGS

Anti-parasitic drugs are used to treat infections caused by various types of parasites, including protozoa, helminths (worms), and ectoparasites like lice and mites. These drugs are typically used under medical supervision to ensure the appropriate treatment of the specific type of parasitic infection. Anti-parasitic drugs are categorized based on the type of parasite they target. Here are the main categories:

Antiprotozoal Agents

Malaria Treatment: Drugs like chloroquine, artemisinin, and mefloquine target Plasmodium species.
Amoebiasis Treatment: Drugs such as metronidazole and tinidazole treat amoebic infections like Entamoeba histolytica.
Giardiasis Treatment: Drugs like metronidazole and tinidazole are used for Giardia infections.
Leishmaniasis Treatment: Amphotericin B, miltefosine, and sodium stibogluconate target Leishmania species.
Trypanosomiasis Treatment: Nifurtimox, benznidazole, and eflornithine treat Trypanosoma infections (e.g., Chagas disease, African sleeping sickness).

Anthelmintic Agents

Nematode (Roundworm) Treatment: Drugs like albendazole, mebendazole, and ivermectin target intestinal and tissue nematodes.
Cestode (Tapeworm) Treatment: Praziquantel and albendazole treat tapeworm infections.
Trematode (Fluke) Treatment: Praziquantel is commonly used against trematode infections, such as schistosomiasis.

Antiectoparasitic Agents

Lice Treatment: Permethrin, malathion, and ivermectin treat lice infestations.

Scabies Treatment: Permethrin and ivermectin are used for scabies caused by Sarcoptes scabiei.
Mite Treatment: Benzyl benzoate and sulfur ointment are sometimes used to treat mite infestations.

Here follows overview of some common anti-parasitic drugs with their brand names and uses.

Albendazole
Treats a variety of parasitic worm infections such as neurocysticercosis (caused by tapeworms), echinococcosis (hydatid disease), ascariasis (roundworm), hookworm, and trichuriasis (whipworm) (*Albenza, Zentel*)

Ivermectin
Effective against a range of parasites, including head lice, scabies, onchocerciasis (river blindness), strongyloidiasis, and other worm infections like ascariasis and filariasis. (*Stromectol, Mectizan, Sklice* - topical for lice)
o
Praziquantel
Used to treat schistosomiasis (a parasitic disease caused by blood flukes), liver flukes, and other flatworm infections such as cysticercosis. (*Biltricide*)
o
Mebendazole
Commonly used to treat intestinal worm infections like pinworm, whipworm, roundworm, and hookworm. (*Vermox, Emverm*)

Metronidazole
Used to treat protozoal infections like giardiasis, amebiasis (Entamoeba histolytica), trichomoniasis, and also for

bacterial infections like bacterial vaginosis. (*Flagyl, Metrogel* - topical)

o

Nitazoxanide
Effective against Giardia lamblia and Cryptosporidium parvum, which cause diarrhea in humans. It also has activity against other protozoa and helminths. (*Alinia*)

o

Permethrin
A topical treatment for head lice and scabies. (*Nix, Elimite*)

Pyrantel Pamoate
Used to treat pinworm, roundworm, and hookworm infections. (*Pin-X, Reese's Pinworm Medicine*)

Tinidazole
Used to treat giardiasis, amebiasis, and trichomoniasis (*Tindamax*)

Diethylcarbamazine
Used for the treatment of lymphatic filariasis, loiasis (African eye worm), and tropical pulmonary eosinophilia. (*Hetrazan*)

ANTIDEPRESSANTS AND ANXIOLYTICS

Antidepressants and anxiolytics are commonly prescribed pharmaceutical drugs used to treat mental health conditions such as depression and anxiety. Alternative health practitioners should have a basic understanding of these medications and how they can be used to complement other holistic treatment modalities.

Antidepressants work by balancing chemicals in the brain called neurotransmitters, which play a key role in regulating mood. They are often prescribed for conditions such as major depressive disorder, generalized anxiety disorder, and obsessive-compulsive disorder. It is important for alternative health practitioners to be aware of the potential side effects and interactions of these medications, as well as the importance of regular monitoring and follow-up with patients.

There are various types of antidepressants.

SSRI (Selective Serotonin Reuptake Inhibitor) Antidepressants

These are mainly used to treat different types of depression. Among them are major depressive disorder and bipolar disorder. Depression's persistent symptoms that last for weeks at time and may be accompanied by physical symptoms, e.g., sleep issues, lack of appetite, and body aches.SSRIs work by increasing the amount of serotonin available in the brain. SSRIs are the first choice of treatment for many types of depression.

Side effects of SSRIs may include dry mouth, diarrhea, nausea, weight gain, vomiting, sexual disorders and poor sleep. Some SSRIs can cause elevated heart rate and the risk for bleeding increases if the patient is using anticoagulants.

Selective serotonin reuptake inhibitor (SSRI)

antidepressants include:

Citalopram (*Celexa*) Fluvoxamine (*Luvox*)
Escitalopram (*Lexapro*) Sertraline (*Zoloft*)
Paroxetine (*Paxil*)

SNRI (Serotonin-norepinephrine reuptake inhibitor) antidepressants

These treat depression but work differently than SSRIs: they work by increasing both Dopamine and Norepinephrine in the brain to improve symptoms. SNRIs might work better in some people if SSRIs haven't brought improvement.

Side effects of SNRIs include are as fro SSRIs. SNRI's can also increase blood pressure and heart rate. Liver function must be monitored in patents on these medications.

SNRI) antidepressants include:

Atomoxetine (*Strattera*)
Duloxetine (*Cymbalta*)
Venlafaxine (*Effexor XR*)
Vesvenlafaxine (*Pristiq*)

MAOI (Mono-Amine Oxidase Inhibitor) antidepressants

These drugs are older antidepressants and aren't widely used today. They're reserved for use when newer medications haven't been effective. MAOIs improve symptoms of depression by increasing dopamine,

norepinephrine, and serotonin levels in the brain.
Side effects of MAOIs may include are as forSSRIs and SNRIs. MAOIs taken with certain foods that have the chemical tyramine can increase blood pressure to dangerous levels.
Tyramine is found in many kinds of cheese, pickles, and some wines.

Monoamine oxidase inhibitor (MAOI) antidepressants include

Isocarboxazid (*Marplan*)
Phenelzine (*Nardil*)
Tranylcypromine (*Parnate*)
Selegiline (*Emsam, Atapryl, Carbex, Eldepryl, Zelapar*)

Tricyclic antidepressants

These are one of the oldest classes of antidepressants still available on the market. They're reserved for use when newer medications haven't been effective. Providers also use tricyclics off-label to treat other conditions. (Off-label use means a drug is used for a condition that doesn't have Food and Drug Administration approval for that condition.)These off-label uses include panic disorder, migraine, chronic pain and obsessive-compulsive disorder. Tricyclics increase the amount of serotonin and norepinephrine in the brain to improve mood.

Side effects of Tricyclics may include those listed for the foregoing categories of antidepressants, and include las weight gain. Additionally, certain groups should avoid tricyclics. This includes people with Glaucoma, heart problems, enlarged prostate, and thyroid issues. These medications can raise blood sugar. In diabetes, it is necessary to carefully monitor sugar levels.

Tricyclic antidepressants include:

Amitriptyline	Imipramine (*Tofranil*)
Amoxapine	Nortriptyline (*Pamelor*)
Desipramine (*Norpramin*)	Protriptyline (*Vivactil*)

Anxiolytics

Anxiolytics, also known as anti-anxiety medications, are used to treat symptoms of anxiety disorders such as panic attacks, social anxiety, and phobias. These medications work by calming the central nervous system and reducing feelings of fear and worry. Alternative health practitioners should be knowledgeable about the different classes of anxiolytics, such as benzodiazepines and SSRIs, and how they can be used safely and effectively in conjunction with other therapies.

When working with patients who are taking antidepressants or anxiolytics, alternative health practitioners should take a collaborative approach with the prescribing physician to ensure the best possible outcomes. This may involve monitoring for potential side effects, discussing any concerns or changes in symptoms, and coordinating care to address the underlying causes of mental health issues. It is also important for practitioners to educate their patients about the importance of adherence to medication regimens and the potential risks of abruptly stopping these medications.

Antidepressants and anxiolytics can be valuable tools in the treatment of mental health conditions when used appropriately and in conjunction with other holistic therapies. Alternative health practitioners should be well-informed about these medications, their mechanisms of action, and how they can be integrated into a comprehensive treatment plan. By working collaboratively with prescribing physicians and providing patient education and support, practitioners can help their patients achieve optimal mental health outcomes.

This drug class is known as benzodiazepines (BZD) They're recommended for short-term use.

BZDs work by increasing GABA levels in the brain, which causes a relaxing or calming effect. They have serious side effects, including dependence and withdrawal.

Side effects of BZDs include:

Dizziness	Loss of balance
Drowsiness	Memory problems
Confusion	Low blood pressure
Depressed breathing	Depressed heart action

This category includes:

Alprazolam (*Xanax*)
Diazepam (*Valium*)
Clonazepam (*Klonopin*)
Lorazepam (*Ativan*)

ANTIPSYCHOTICS

Antipsychotic drugs, also known as neuroleptics, are a class of medications primarily used to treat psychiatric disorders such as schizophrenia, bipolar disorder, and severe depression. These drugs work by blocking certain neurotransmitters in the brain, specifically dopamine, which helps to reduce symptoms of psychosis, hallucinations, and delusions. While antipsychotics can be incredibly effective in managing these conditions, they also come with a range of potential side effects that must be carefully monitored.

One of the most common side effects of antipsychotic medications is weight gain. Many patients who take these drugs find that they experience significant increases in appetite and may gain weight rapidly. This can be particularly concerning for individuals who are already struggling with their mental health, as weight gain can exacerbate feelings of low self-esteem and body image issues. Alternative health practitioners should work closely with their patients to monitor their weight and provide guidance on healthy eating habits and exercise routines to mitigate this side effect.

Another important consideration when prescribing antipsychotics is the risk of metabolic syndrome. This condition is characterized by a cluster of symptoms including high blood pressure, high blood sugar levels, and abnormal cholesterol levels. Patients taking antipsychotic medications are at an increased risk of developing metabolic syndrome, which can lead to serious health complications such as heart disease and diabetes. Alternative health practitioners should monitor their patients closely for signs of metabolic syndrome and work with them to make lifestyle changes that can reduce their risk.

In addition to physical side effects, antipsychotic medications can also have a significant impact on a patient's mental health. Some individuals may experience feelings of sedation, lethargy, or cognitive impairment while taking these drugs. It is important for alternative health practitioners to closely monitor their patients for any changes in mood or behavior that could indicate a negative reaction to the medication. Adjustments to the dosage or type of antipsychotic may be necessary to ensure the patient's well-being.

Overall, antipsychotic medications can be a valuable tool in the treatment of psychiatric disorders, but they must be used carefully and monitored closely to minimize potential side effects. Alternative health practitioners should work closely with their patients to educate them about the risks and benefits of these medications and develop a comprehensive treatment plan that addresses both their mental and physical health needs. By taking a holistic approach to prescribing antipsychotics, practitioners can help their patients achieve optimal outcomes and improve their overall quality of life.

Antipsychotic medications may be classified as typical, atypical, mood stabilizers and stimulants.

Typical antipsychotics

These drugs treat symptoms associated with schizophrenia. They may also be used for other conditions. The first antipsychotic drug in this class, chlorpromazine, was introduced more than 60 years ago and is still in use. Typical antipsychotics block dopamine in the brain. Side effects of antipsychotic drugs include:

Blurred vision
Nausea
Vomiting
Trouble sleeping

Anxiety
Drowsiness
Weight gain
Sexual problems

This class of drugs causes movement-related disorders called extrapyramidal side effects, specifically tardive dyskenisia (TDK).

Typical antipsychotics include:

Chlorpromazine (*Thorazine*)
Fluphenazine (*Prolixin*)
Haloperidol (*Haldol*)
Perphenazine (*Trilafon*)
Thioridazine (*Mellaril*)

Atypical antipsychotics

These are the next generation, the most recently developed of medications used to treat schizophrenia. These drugs work by blocking brain chemicals dopamine D2 and serotonin 5-HT2A receptor activity. Physicians also use atypical antipsychotics to treat symptoms of Bipolar disorder, Depression and Tourette syndrome.

Atypical antipsychotics have some serious side effects including an increased risk of diabetes, high cholesterol levels, heart muscle–related problems, involuntary movements, including muscle spasms, tremors and stroke. Aripiprazole (Abilify), clozapine (Clozaril), and quetiapine (Seroquel) have a black box warning for specific safety concerns. There's a risk of suicidal thoughts and behaviors in people under the age of 18 who take one of these medications.

Side effects of atypical antipsychotics include:

Dizziness	Constipation
Dry mouth	Weight gain
Blurred vision	Sleepiness

Atypical antipsychotics include:

Aripiprazole (*Abilify*)	Paliperidone (*Invega*)
Clozapine (*Clozaril*)	Quetiapine (*Seroquel*)
Iloperidone (*Fanapt*)	Risperidone (*Risperdal*)
Olanzapine (*Zyprexa*)	Ziprasidone (*Geodon*)

Mood stabilizers

Mood stabilizers use these drugs to treat depression and other mood disorders, like bipolar disorder. The exact way mood stabilizers work isn't well understood yet. Some researchers believe these medications calm specific areas of the brain that contribute to the mood changes of bipolar disorder and related conditions. Side effects of mood stabilizers may include:

Dizziness	Nausea
Vomiting	Tiredness
Stomach problems	

The kidneys remove lithium (contained in these medications) from the body,
so kidney function and levels of lithium must be regularly checked. If poor
kidney function results, providers may need to adjust the dose.

Mood stabilizers include:

Carbamazepine (*Carbatrol, Tegretol, Tegretol XR*)
Divalproex sodium (*Depakote*)
Lamotrigine (*Lamictal*)
Lithium (*Eskalith, Eskalith CR, Lithobid*)

Stimulants

These drugs mainly treat attention deficit hyperactivity disorder (ADHD). Stimulants increase dopamine and norepinephrine in the brain. The body can develop dependence if used long term.

Side effects of stimulants include problems with sleep, poor appetite, weight loss. Stimulants can increase heart rate and blood pressure. They may not be an appropriate option if there are heart or blood pressure problems. Stimulants include:

Amphetamine (*Adderall, Adderall XR*)
Dexmethylphenidate (*Focalin, Focalin XR*)
Dextroamphetamine (*Dexedrine*)
Lisdexamfetamine (*Vyvanse*)
Methylphenidate (*Ritalin, Metadate ER, Methylin, Concerta*)

CARDIAC DRUGS

Cardiac drugs include Statins, Antiplatelet (*Clopidogrel*), Anticoagulants, Beta Blockers, Calcium channel blockers (CCBs), and ACE Inhibitors Cardiovascular agents are medicines that are used to treat medical conditions associated with the heart or the circulatory system (blood vessels), such as arrhythmias, blood clots, coronary artery disease, high or low blood pressure, high cholesterol, heart failure, and stroke.

Some of the major types of commonly prescribed cardiovascular medications are elaborated in this section. For your information and reference, I have included generic names as well as major trade names to help identify what you or your patient may be taking.

It is important to be aware of potential drug interactions with antihypertensive medications. Some medications, such as nonsteroidal anti-inflammatory drugs (NSAIDs) and certain antidepressants, can interfere with the effectiveness of antihypertensives. It is important to review patients' medication lists carefully and consult with other healthcare providers as needed to ensure that there are no interactions that could compromise the effectiveness of the antihypertensive therapy. By staying informed and vigilant, alternative health practitioners can provide the best possible care for their patients with hypertension.

Anticoagulants

Anticoagulants (Also known as Blood Thinners) decrease the clotting (coagulating) ability of the blood. They are sometimes called blood thinners, although they do not actually thin the blood. They do NOT dissolve existing blood clots, and are used to treat certain blood vessel, heart and lung conditions.

They are ordinarily prescribed:

    To prevent harmful clots from forming in the blood vessels.
    To prevent the clots from becoming larger and causing more serious problems.
    To prevent first or recurrent strokes.

Commonly prescribed anticoagulants include:

    Apixaban (*Eliquis*)
    Dabigatran (*Pradaxa*)
    Edoxaban (*Savaysa*)
    Heparin (various)
    Rivaroxaban (*Xarelto*)
    Warfarin (*Coumadin*)

Antiplatelet Agents

Antiplatelet Agents Keeps blood clots from forming by preventing blood platelets from sticking together. Commonly prescribed antiplatelet agents are used::

    To prevent clotting in patients who have had a heart attack, unstable angina, ischemic strokes, transient ischemic attacks (TIA) and other forms of cardiovascular disease.

To prevent plaque buildup is evident but there is not yet a major blockage in the artery.

Certain patients will be prescribed aspirin combined with another antiplatelet drug – also known as dual antiplatelet therapy (DAPT).

Commonly prescribed include:

>Acetylsalicylic Acid (*Aspirin)*
>Clopidogrel (*Plavix*)
>Dipyridamole (*Persantine*)
>Prasugrel (*Effient*)
>Ticagrelor (*Brilinta*)

ACE Inhibitors/Anti-Hypertensives

Angiotensin Converting Enzyme (ACE) inhibitors expand blood vessels and decrease resistance by lowering levels of angiotensin II. This allows blood to flow more easily and makes the heart's work easier and more efficient.

ACE inhibitors are commonly used to treat or improve symptoms of cardiovascular conditions including high blood pressure and heart failure.
Commonly prescribed include:

Benazepril (*Lotensin*)
Captopril (*Capoten*)
Enalapril (Vasotec)
Lisinopril (*Prinivil, Zestril*)
Moexipril (*Univasc*)
Ramipril (*Altace*)
Trandolapril (*Mavik*)

ARB Inhibitors/Anti-Hypertensives

Angiotensin II Receptor Blockers or Inhibitors (also known as ARBs), rather than lowering levels of angiotensin II (as ACE inhibitors do) prevent this chemical from having any effect on the heart and blood vessels. This keeps blood pressure from rising.
ARBs are commonly Used to treat or improve symptoms of cardiovascular conditions including high blood pressure and heart failure.
Commonly ARBs prescribed include:

- Azilsartan (*Edarbi*)
- Candesartan (*Atacand*)
- Eprosartan (*Teveten*)
- Irbesartan (*Avapro*)
- Losartan (*Cozaar*)
- Olmesartan (*Benicar*)
- Telmisartan (*Micardis*)
- Valsartan (*Diovan*)

ARN Inhibitors/Anti-Hypertensives

Angiotensin Receptor-Neprilysin Inhibitors (ARNIs) are a drug combination of a neprilysin inhibitor and an ARB. Neprilysin is an enzyme that breaks down natural substances in the body that open narrowed arteries.

By limiting the effect of neprilysin, it increases the effects of these substances and improves artery opening and blood flow, reduces sodium (salt) retention, and decreases strain on the heart. ARNIs are commonly prescribed along with an ARB Inhibitor (e.g., Valsartan) for the treatment of heart failure.

Commonly prescribed ARNIs include:

Sacubitril (*Entresto*)

Beta Blockers / Anti-Hypertensives/Anti-Arrythmics

Also known as Beta-Adrenergic Blocking Agents), Beta blockers decrease the heart rate and force of contraction, which lowers blood pressure and makes the heart beat more slowly and with less force.

Beta blockers are commonly prescribed to:
>To lower blood pressure.
>For cardiac arrhythmias (abnormal heart rhythms)
>To treat chest pain (angina)
>To help prevent future heart attacks in patients who have had a heart attack.

Commonly prescribed Beta blockers include:

>Acebutolol (*Sectral*)
>Atenolol (*Tenormin*)
>Bisoprolol/hydrochlorothiazide (*Ziac*)
>Bisoprolol (*Zebeta*)
>Metoprolol (*Lopressor, Toprol XL*)
>Nadolol (*Corgard*)
>Propranolol (*Inderal*)
>Sotalol (*Betapace*)

Calcium Blockers / Anti-Hypertensives

Calcium Blockers (also known as Calcium Antagonists or Calcium Channel Blockers) interrupt the movement of

calcium into the cells of the heart and blood vessels. They may decrease the heart's pumping strength and relax blood vessels.
Calcium blockers are commonly prescribed to treat high blood pressure, chest pain (angina) caused by reduced blood supply to the heart muscle and some arrhythmias (abnormal heart rhythms).

Commonly prescribed include:

Amlodipine (*Norvasc*)
    Diltiazem (*Cardizem, Tiazac*)
    Felodipine (*Plendil*)
    Nifedipine (*Adalat, Procardia*)
    Nimodipine (Nimotop)
    Nisoldipine (*Sular*)
    Verapamil (*Calan, Verelan*)

Statins

The premier group of Cholesterol-lowering medications consists of the Statins. Other drugs are sometimes used by individuals who suffer severe side effects from Statins or in whom they are ineffective, and these include nicotinic acids, niacin, cholesterol absorption inhibitor such as Ezetimibe (Zetia) but these are infrequently used. Statins, also known as HMG-CoA reductase inhibitors, reduce illness and mortality in those who are at high risk of cardiovascular disease and are the most common cholesterol-lowering drugs.

Statins are used to lower LDL cholesterol.

Commonly used Statin include:

Atorvastatin (*Lipitor*)
Fluvastatin (*Lescol*)
Lovastatin (*Mevacor*)
Pitavastatin (*Livalo*)
Pravastatin (*Pravachol*)
Rosuvastatin (*Crestor*)
Simvastatin (*Zocor*)

Digitalis Preparations

Digitalis Preparations Increase the force of the heart's contractions and can be beneficial in treating heart failure and irregular heartbeats.

They are commonly used to relieve heart failure symptoms, especially when the patient isn't responding to other standard treatments including ACE inhibitors, ARBs and diuretics. They also slow certain types of irregular heartbeat (arrhythmias), particularly atrial fibrillation.

Commonly used Digitalis preparations include:

*   Digoxin (*Lanoxin*)

Diuretics / Anti-Hypertensives

Diuretics (also known as water pills) cause the body to rid itself of excess fluids and sodium through urination and thus helps to reduce the heart's workload. They also decrease the buildup of fluid in the lungs and other parts of the body, e.g., the ankles and legs. Diuretics remove fluid at varied rates and through different methods.

They are commonly used:to help lower blood pressure and to help reduce swelling (edema) from excess buildup of fluid in the body.

Commonly prescribed include:

- Acetazolamide (*Diamox*)
- Amiloride (*Midamor*)
- Bumetanide (*Bumex*)
- Chlorothiazide (*Diuril*)
- Chlorthalidone (*Hygroton*)
- Furosemide (*Lasix*)
- Hydro-chlorothiazide (*Esidrix, Hydrodiuril*)
- Indapamide (*Lozol*)
- Metalozone (*Zaroxolyn*)
- Spironolactone (*Aldactone*)
- Torsemide (*Demadex*)

Vasodilators

Vasodilators relax blood vessels and decreases blood pressure. The largest and most important category of vasodilators called nitrates increases the supply of blood and oxygen to the heart while reducing its workload which can ease chest pain (angina). Nitroglycerin, one widely used vasodilator, is available as a pill to be swallowed or (absorbed under the tongue (sublingual), a spray, and as a topical application (cream).

These are prescribed to relieve chest pain (angina pectoris).Commonly prescribed Vasodilators include:

- Isosorbide dinitrate (*Isordil*)
- Isosorbide mononitrate (*Imdur*)

Hydralazine (*Apresoline*)
Nitroglycerin (*Nitro Bid, Nitro Stat*)

RESPIRATORY AGENTS

Respiratory agents include Bronchodilators (short-term and long-term Beta Agonists), Racemic Epinephrine, Corticosteroids, and Mucolytics, Cough Suppressants and Expectorants.
These include a wide variety of medicines used to relieve, treat, or prevent respiratory diseases such as asthma, chronic bronchitis, chronic obstructive pulmonary disease (COPD), or pneumonia.

Respiratory agents are available in many different forms, such as oral tablets, oral liquids, injections or inhalations.

Bronchodilators

A bronchodilator or broncholytic (although the latter occasionally includes secretory inhibition as well) is a substance that dilates the bronchi and bronchioles, decreasing resistance in the respiratory airway and increasing airflow to the lungs. Bronchodilators may be originating naturally within the body, or they may be medications administered for the treatment of breathing difficulties. Bronchodilators are either short-acting or long-acting. Short-acting medications provide quick or "rescue" relief from acute bronchoconstriction. Long-acting bronchodilators help to control and prevent symptoms.

The three types of prescription bronchodilating drugs are

beta2-adrenergic agonists (short- and long-acting), anticholinergics (short- and long-acting), and theophylline (long-acting).

Short acting: These are quick-relief or "rescue" medications that provide quick, temporary relief from asthma symptoms or flare-ups. These medications (e.g., *Salbutamol*) usually take effect within 20 minutes or less, and can last from four to six hours. These inhaled medications are best for treating sudden and severe or new asthma symptoms.

Long acting: taken routinely in order to control and prevent bronchoconstriction. They are not intended for fast relief. These medications (e.g., *Salmeterol*) may take longer to begin working, but relieve airway constriction for up to 12 hours. Commonly taken twice a day with an anti-inflammatory medication, they maintain open airways and prevent asthma symptoms, particularly at night.

Another category of bronchodilators is anticholinergics (e.g., Spiriva (tiotropium). These are long-acting, 24-hour, bronchodilators used in the management of chronic obstructive pulmonary disease (COPD). They are only available as inhalants.

As a short-acting anticholinergic, they improves lung function and reduces the risk of exacerbation in people with symptomatic asthma. However, they will not stop an asthma attack already in progress. Because they has no effect on asthma symptoms when used alone, they are most often paired with a short-acting beta- agonist. While it is considered a relief or rescue medication, it can take a full hour to begin working. For this reason, it plays a secondary role in acute asthma treatment.

A further category of bronchodilators is theophylline, available in oral and injectable form, is a long-acting bronchodilator that prevents asthma episodes. It is prescribed in severe cases of asthma or those that are difficult to control. It must be taken 1–4 times daily, and doses cannot be missed. Blood tests are required to monitor therapy and to indicate when dosage adjustment is necessary.
Side effects can include nausea, vomiting, diarrhea, stomach or headache, rapid or irregular heartbeat, muscle cramps, nervous or jittery feelings, and hyperactivity. These symptoms may signal the need for an adjustment in medication. It may promote acid reflux, also known as GERD, by relaxing the lower esophageal sphincter muscle. Many other medications cross-react with Theophylline.

Short-acting bronchodilators include:
    Salbutamol/albuterol (*Proventil* or *Ventolin*)
    Levosalbutamol/levalbuterol (*Xopenex*)
    Pirbuterol (*Maxair*)
    Epinephrine (*Primatene Mist*)
    Racemic Epinephrine (*Asthmanefrin, Primatene Mist* Replacement)
    Ephedrine (*Bronkaid*)
    Terbutaline (*Brethine*)
Long-acting bronchodilators include:

Salmeterol (*Serevent* or *Seretide*)
Clenbuterol (*Spiropent*)
Formoterol (*Forodil, Perforomist*)

Bambuterol (*Bambec*)
Indacaterol (*Arcapta*)
Theophylline (*Theo-24, Elixophyllin, Theolair ER*)

Racemic Epinephrine

Racemic Epinephrine is used for temporary relief of symptoms associated with bronchial asthma (e.g., shortness of breath, chest tightening, wheezing) in adults and children and to treat croup in children. Racemic epinephrine is an inhaled bronchodilator that is made from both a bronchodilator and epinephrine mixed together. The medications together to help reduce the inflammation in the airways. The bronchodilator opens up the airways and the epinephrine helps to keep them open. The epinephrine is also a powerful anti-histamine that helps reduce reactions to certain chemicals in the body that produce the inflammation in the lungs.

It is available under the brand names *AsthmaNefrin* and *S2*.

It is administered via nebulized solution, and is available in both over-the-counter and prescription strengths.

Corticosteroids

Inhaled corticosteroids act directly in the lungs to inhibit the inflammatory process that causes asthma. Inhaled corticosteroids help to prevent asthma attacks and improve lung function. They may also be used in the treatment of certain other lung conditions, such as chronic obstructive pulmonary disease (COPD). These are all in a preparation designed to be inhaled through the mouth

Inhaled corticosteroids contain corticosteroids such as:

beclomethasone,
budesonide,
ciclesonide,
flunisolide,
fluticasone,
mometasone

Inhaled corticosteroids act directly in the lungs and because inhaled corticosteroids deliver the medicine directly into the lungs, much smaller doses of corticosteroid are needed to effectively control asthma symptoms compared to what would be needed if the same medication was taken orally. This also reduces the likelihood of side effects.

These include:

>*Flovent*
>*Qvar Redi-haler*
>*Alvesco*
>*Asmanex Twisthaler*
>*Pulmicort Respules*
>*Arnuity, Elipta*
>*Aerospan*
>*Aerobid*
>*Becloven*

Mucolytics

Overproduction of mucus in the lungs—usually seen with COPD or sometimes with a lower respiratory infection—is caused by inflammation that results in an increase in both the number and size of so-called goblet cells that line the air passages.

While goblet cells normally secrete mucus as a form of protection, with COPD, for example, the excessive production can clog the passages, making it harder to breathe. One way of clearing this buildup is with an oral or nebulized drug called a mucolytics.
Mucolytic agents are able to alter the secretion of mucus and its physical properties which results in improvement of mucociliary clearance.

Mucolyrics include:

- Erdosteine (*MucoMyst, Acys-5*)
- Mecysteine (*Mucinex* [guaifenesin])
  Bromhexine (*Bisolvon, Axcel, Barkicin*)
  Pulmozyme (*Dornase Alfa*)

Cough Suppressants and Expectorants

Cough suppressants and expectorants are two commonly used types of pharmaceutical drugs in the treatment of respiratory conditions. Alternative health practitioners often incorporate these medications into their treatment plans to help their patients manage coughing symptoms effectively. Understanding the differences between cough suppressants and expectorants is crucial for providing the best care possible to patients.

Cough suppressants work by blocking the cough reflex in the brain, reducing the urge to cough. This can be helpful in situations where a persistent cough is causing discomfort or interfering with daily activities. Common ingredients found in cough suppressants include *dextromethorphan* and *codeine*. It is important to note that cough suppressants should not be used for productive coughs, as they can prevent the body from clearing mucus from the lungs.

On the other hand, expectorants work by loosening mucus in the airways, making it easier to cough up. This can be beneficial for patients with chest congestion or a productive cough. *Guaifenesin* is a common ingredient found in expectorants, and it is often used to help thin and loosen mucus in the respiratory tract. Alternative health practitioners may recommend expectorants to help their patients clear mucus from their lungs and improve breathing.

When choosing between cough suppressants and expectorants, alternative health practitioners must consider the specific symptoms and needs of their patients. It is important to assess whether the patient has a dry, non-productive cough that would benefit from a cough suppressant, or a chesty, productive cough that would benefit from an expectorant. By tailoring their treatment plans to the individual needs of each patient, alternative health practitioners can provide more effective care and support.

Cough suppressants and expectorants are valuable tools in the management of respiratory conditions. Alternative health practitioners can use these medications to help their patients alleviate coughing symptoms and improve their overall quality of life. By understanding the differences between these two types of medications and selecting the most appropriate option for each patient, alternative health practitioners can effectively incorporate pharmaceutical remedies into their treatment plans.

ENDOCRINE DRUGS

This category includes Adrenal drugs, Anabolic steroids, Androgens, Antiandrogens, Antidiabetics, Calcitropic vitamins & minerals, Estrogen, Obesity drugs, Progesterone, and Thyroid Agents. Endocrine drugs can be natural (from animals), semi- synthetic, or synthetic compounds Endocrine drugs are agents directed to a malfunctioning endocrine path. Several agents are secreted in or target the nervous system, and are thus more prone to cause neurologic adverse events (AEs). This chapter focuses on commonly used endocrine agents directed to the hypothalamus-pituitary axis, thyroid, and antidiabetic agents.

The use of drugs to help regulate and control endocrine function is an important area of pharmacology. In one sense, hormones can be considered drugs that are manufactured by the patient's body. This situation presents an obvious opportunity to use exogenous chemicals to either mimic or attenuate the effects of specific hormones during endocrine dysfunction, i.e, where those naturally proceed hormones are either lacking or present in over-abundance.

Anabolic Steroids

Anabolic steroids are synthetic, or human-made, variations of the male sex hormone testosterone. The proper term for these compounds is anabolic-androgenic steroids. "Anabolic" refers to muscle building, and "androgenic" refers to increased male sex characteristics. Anabolic steroids include all synthetic derivatives of testosterone, both oral and injectable.

Examples of anabolic steroids include testosterone, methyltestosterone, danazol, and oxandrolone.

Health care providers use anabolic steroids to treat some hormone problems in men, such as delayed puberty. They are also used for gaining body mass from more protein production in the body, lowering your overall body fat percentage, gaining muscle strength and endurance, increasing bones density (osteoporosis), increasing red blood cell production (anemia) and maintaining muscle mass with conditions like endometriosis, liver disease or cancer that causes muscles to waste away and underweight in infants.

Commercially available prescribed anabolic steroids include *Testosterone, Primobolan, Anavar, Deca Durabolin* and *Dianabol*. In the U.S. they are classified as Schedule III Controlled Substances due to the possibility of serious adverse effects and a high potential for abuse.

Androgens

Androgens, a particular subset of steroids, are a group of hormones that play a role in the development male traits and reproductive activity. Present in both males and females, the principle androgens are *testosterone* and *androstenedione.* Androgens may be called "male hormones," but are present in both male and female bodies in differing amounts. Hormones created from cholesterol, like androgens and estrogen, are known as *steroid hormones.*

Androgens play a role insulin sensitivity, and also impact bone density and cardiovascular health in cisgender females, and *may* have an impact on brain function and mood.

The most "important" estrogen, *estradiol*, is actually synthesized from testosterone by an enzyme called *aromatase.* Androgens also appear to impact the function of the endometrium (the lining of the uterus), and may play a role in helping prepare it to support a potential pregnancy.

There are few symptoms of low androgen levels in females, but in males lower than optimal levels may be accompanied by diabetes, the development of thyroid problems, high blood pressure, high cholesterol, depression and anxiety.

Antiandrogens

Antiandrogens, also known as androgen antagonists or testosterone blockers, are a class of drugs that prevent androgens like testosterone, androstenedione, and dihydrotestosterone (DHT) from mediating their biological effects in the body. They act by blocking the androgen receptor (AR) and/or inhibiting or suppressing androgen production.

Antiandrogens are used in the treatment of various conditions and disorders including prostate cancer, precocious puberty in young males, benign prostatic hyperplasia, androgenic alopecia (male-pattern hair loss) and sexual disorders, such as hyper-sexuality, in men.

In women, antiandrogens may be used to treat polycystic ovary syndrome, hirsutism (excessive facial or body hair), amenorrhea (absence of menstrual periods), acne, and several other conditions.

Available antiandrogens include:

>Enzalutamide (*Xtandi*)
>Bicalutamide (*Casodex*)
>Apalutamide (*Erleqda*)
>Darolutamide (*Nubeqa*)
>Nilutamide (*Nilandron*)
>Flutamide (*Eulexin*)

Anti-Diabetic Drugs

Antidiabetic drug, any drug that works to lower abnormally high glucose (sugar) levels in the blood, which are characteristic of the endocrine system disorder known as diabetes mellitus. Diabetes is caused by the bodys inability to produce or respond to the pancreatic hormone insulin. A number of generic and branded antidiabetic drugs fall under these types.

Anti-diabetic drugs can be categorized into the following classes:

A. Metformin

B. Sulfonureas
C. Glinides
D. Thiazolidinediones
E. DPP-4 inhibitors
F. GLP-1 receptor agonists
G. SGLT2 inhibitors
H. Insulin

Each act to control diabetes in its own way, and each s optimal for a variety of diabetic patients.

Metformin (*Fortamet, Glumetza*, others) is generally the first medication prescribed for type 2 diabetes. It works primarily by lowering glucose production in the liver and improving your body's sensitivity to insulin so that your body uses insulin more effectively.
Some people experience B-12 deficiency and may need to take supplements. Other possible side effects, which may improve over time, include Nausea, Abdominal pain, Bloating, and Diarrhea.

Sulfonylureas help your body secrete more insulin. Examples include glyburide (*DiaBeta, Glynase*), glipizide (*Glucotrol*) and glimepiride (*Amaryl*). Possible side effects include Low blood sugar (hypoglycemia) and Weight gain

Glinides stimulate the pancreas to secrete more insulin. They're faster acting than sulfonylureas, and the duration of their effect in the body is shorter. Examples include repaglinide and nateglinide. Possible side effects include Low blood sugar (hypoglycemia) and weight gain.

Thiazolidinediones make the body's tissues more sensitive to insulin. Examples include rosiglitazone (*Avandia*) and pioglitazone (*Actos*). Possible side effects include Risk of congestive heart failure, Risk of bladder cancer (pioglitazone), Risk of bone fractures, High cholesterol (rosiglitazone) and Weight gain

DPP-4 inhibitors help reduce blood sugar levels but tend to have a very modest effect. Examples include sitagliptin (*Januvia*), saxagliptin (*Onglyza*) and linagliptin (*Tradjenta*). Possible side effects include risk of pancreatitis, Joint pain

GLP-1 receptor agonists are injectable medications that slow digestion and help lower blood sugar levels. Their use is often associated with weight loss (and are often used off-label for that purpose), and some may reduce the risk of heart attack and stroke. Examples include exenatide (*Byetta, Bydureon*), liraglutide (*Saxenda, Victoza*) and semaglutide (*Rybelsus, Ozempic*) and Tirzepatide (*Mounjouro*). Possible side effects include risk of pancreatitis, nausea, vomiting, diarrhea.

SGLT2 inhibitors affect the blood-filtering functions in your kidneys by inhibiting the return of glucose to the bloodstream. As a result, glucose is excreted in the urine. These drugs may reduce the risk of heart attack and stroke in people with a high risk of those conditions. Examples include canagliflozin (*Invokana*), dapagliflozin (*Farxiga*) and empagliflozin (*Jardiance*). Possible side effects include: Risk of amputation (canagliflozin), Risk of bone fractures (canagliflozin), Risk of gangrene, Vaginal yeast infections, Urinary tract infections, Low blood pressure and High cholesterol

Other medications include blood pressure and cholesterol-lowering medications, as well as low-dose aspirin, to help prevent heart and blood vessel disease.

Some people who have type 2 diabetes need *insulin* therapy. In the past, insulin therapy was used as a last resort, but today it may be prescribed sooner if blood sugar targets aren't met with lifestyle changes and other medications. Side effects of insulin include the risk of low blood sugar (hypoglycemia), diabetic ketoacidosis and high triglycerides.

Calcitropic Hormones

Calcitropic hormone is general term for any hormone (e.g., calcitonin or PTH) which plays a major role in bone growth and remodelling. The endocrine factors involved in calcium are known as calciotropic hormones and include calcitonin, parathyroid hormone (PTH), 1,25-dihydroxyvitamin D3 (that is, active vitamin D), and fibroblast growth factor 23 (FGF23).

The main actions of calcitonin are to increase bone calcium content and decrease the blood calcium level when it rises above normal. Calcitonin also lowers blood phosphorus levels when they rise above normal.

If calcitonin levels are high, it may mean suggest C-cell hyperplasia or medullary thyroid cancer.

There is a progressive decrease of plasma calcitonin with age. Postmenopausal females have a significantly smaller calcitonin reserve, leaving them at risk of osteoporosis. Thus, Calcitonin injection is used to treat osteoporosis in postmenopausal women.

Calcitonin injection is also used to treat Paget's disease of bone and to quickly reduce calcium levels in the blood (enhancing its transfer to bone tissue or its excretion) when needed.

Estrogen

Estrogen or oestrogen, is a category of sex hormone responsible for the development and regulation of the female reproductive system and secondary sex characteristics.
There are three major endogenous estrogens that have estrogenic hormonal activity: estrone (E1), estradiol (E2), and estriol (E3).
Estradiol is the most potent and prevalent.
Estrogen is responsible for the development and regulation of the female reproductive system and secondary sex characteristics.
In addition to their role as natural hormones, estrogens are used as medications:
mainly in hormonal contraception, post-meopausal hormone replacement therapy, or as a feminizing therapy in gender dysphoria and transgendered individual.

Progesterone

Progesterone is an endogenous steroid and progestogen sex hormone involved in the menstrual cycle, pregnancy, and embryogenesis of humans and other species.
It belongs to a group of steroid hormones called the progestogens and is the major progestogen in the body.

Progesterone has a variety of important functions in the body. Progesterone is also used as a medication, such as in combination with estrogen for contraception, to reduce the risk of uterine or cervical cancer, in hormone replacement therapy, and in feminizing hormone therapy.

Progesterone has been shown to prevent miscarriage in women with vaginal bleeding early in their current pregnancy and a previous history of miscarriage. Progesterone can be taken by mouth, through the vagina, and by injection into muscle or fat.

Obesity Drugs

Obesity is a chronic disease that affects more than 4 in 10 adults in the United States, and nearly 1 in 10 Americans have severe obesity. Prescription medications to treat overweight and obesity work in different ways. For example, some medications may help diminish awareness of hunger while other medications may make it harder for the body to absorb fat from foods eaten.

Xenical (orlistat) works in your gut to reduce the amount of fat the body absorbs from food.
Available in lower dose without prescription, it may be used by adults and children ages 12 and older. Common side effects include diarrhea, gas, leakage of oily stools and stomach pain.
Rare cases of severe liver injury have been reported. There is a major cross-reaction with Cyclosporine.

Qsymia (phentermine-topiramate) is a mix of two medications: phentermine, which lessens the appetite, and topiramate, which is used to treat seizures and migraine headaches.

It should be used only be adults. The net effect is that it diminishes the sense of hunger and increases satiation. Common side effects include constipation, dizziness, dry mouth, taste changes (especially with carbonated beverages), tingling of the hands and feet and insomnia. *Qsymia* should not be used in persons with glaucoma or hyperthyroidism, who have or had a heart attack or stroke, abnormal heart rhythm, kidney disease, or mood level issues.It should not be taken during or just before pregnancy (it has caused birth defects) or while breastfeeding

Contrave (naltrexone-bupropion) is a mixture of two medications: naltrexone, which is used to treat alcohol and drug dependence, and bupropion, which is used to treat depression or help smoking cessation, and should only be used by adults.It allays the sensation of hunger and promotes satiation .Common side effects are constipation, diarrhea, dizziness, dry mouth, headache, increased blood pressure, increased heart rate, insomnia, liver damage, and nausea and vomiting. It should not be used in patients with uncontrolled high blood pressure, seizures, or a history of anorexia or bulimia nervosa, who are dependent on opioid pain medications or are withdrawing from drugs or alcohol or who are taking bupropion (*Wellbutrin, Zyban*).*Contrave* may cause or amplify suicidal thoughts or actions.

Saxenda (liraglutide) is given daily by injection and may be used by adults and children ages 12 years and older. *Saxenda* mimics a hormone called glucagon-like peptide-1 (GLP-1) that targets areas of the brain that regulate appetite and food intake, diminishing appetite and increasing satiation. Common side effects include nausea, diarrhea, constipation, abdominal pain, headache, and increased heart rate. *Saxenda* may increase the chance of developing pancreatitis, and has been found to cause a rare type of thyroid tumor in animals.

Wegovy (semaglutide) iis given weekly by injection to adults. It mimics a hormone called glucagon-like peptide-1 (GLP-1) that targets areas of the brain that regulate appetite and food intake. Common side effects include nausea, diarrhea, vomiting, constipation, abdominal (stomach) pain, headache, and fatigue. *Wegovy* should not be used in combination with other semaglutide-containing products, other GLP-1 receptor agonists, or other products intended for weight loss, including prescription drugs, over-the-counter drugs, or herbal products. It may increase the chance of developing pancreatitis and as been found to cause a rare type of thyroid tumor in animals.

Imcivree (setmelanotide) is available by injection only and only to patients ages 6 years and older with obesity due to three specific rare genetic conditions. It reduces appetite and increases feeling of fullness and may increase resting metabolism. Although it can help the patient lose weight, it does not treat the causative genetic defects Common side effects include injection site reaction, skin darkening, nausea, disturbance in sexual arousal, depression and suicidal ideation, and a risk of serious adverse reactions in neonates and infants with low birthweight, owing to the benzyl alcohol preservative. *Imcivree* is intended only for people with any of these extremely rare genetic diseases, confirmed by genetic testing:

POMC (proopiomelanocortin) deficiency, PCSK1 (proprotein convertase subtilisin/kexin type 1) deficiency or LEPR (leptin receptor) deficiency. Not for use while pregnant or breastfeeding.

Other Anti-Obesity Drugs: Other medications that curb appetite include:

>Phentermine
>Benzphetamine
>Diethylpropion
>Phendimetrazine

It should be noted that some antidiabetic drugs are given an off-label use for weigth control, notably *Ozempic* and *Monjouro*

These are for use by adults and are FDA-approved only for short-term use—up to 12 weeks. They act by Increasing brain chemicals diminishing awareness of hunger and promoting satiation. They should not be used by persons having heart disease, uncontrolled high blood pressure, hyperthyroidism, or glaucoma. Possible side effects include dry mouth, constipation, difficulty sleeping, dizziness, nervousness, restlessness, headache, heightened blood pressure and an increased heart rate.

Thyroid Agents

Thyroid drugs (thyroid hormones) are used to supplement low thyroid levels in people with hypothyroidism.

Hypothyroidism is a condition in which the thyroid gland does not produce enough thyroid hormones to meet the needs of the body, which may result from a disease condition or from surgical removal of th thyroid gland. Even though thyroid hormones are made in the thyroid gland, the production of these hormones is regulated by another hormone, called thyroid stimulating hormone (TSH), which is made by the pituitary gland

Another condition, called hyperthyroidism, is when the thyroid produces too much thyroid hormone. Although hyperthyroidism seems to be the opposite of hypothyroidism, the link between them is complex, and one can lead to the other in certain circumstances. Hyperthyroidism is often treated surgically. Hypothyroidism is treated by augmentation with thyroid hormone.

There are natural preparations are derived from animal thyroid tissue: these include desiccated thyroid and thyroglobulin. However, the most common thyroid medication is synthetic thyroxine, also known by the name of Levothyroxine . *Liotrix* is another commonly used thyroid medication.

Commonly used thyroid drugs include: Levothyroxin and Liothyronine sold under brand names as *Synthroid, Cytomel, Tirosint, Triostat Euthyrox, Levoxyl, Liotrix, Unithroid, Tyrolar, Levothroid, Levo-T,* and *Thyrotopin Alpha.*

Dissicated thyroid gland is sold under he brand names *Armour Thyroid, NP Thyroid, Naturthroid* and *Westhroid.*

IMMUNOLOGIC AGENTS

Immunologic agents are drugs that can modify the immune response, either by enhancing or suppressing the immune system. They are used to fight infections, prevent and treat certain diseases.

Immunologic agents include drugs used for immunosuppression to prevent graft rejection. They can be used as cancer chemotherapy agents. Some immunologic agents can down-regulate the inflammatory process and can be used to treat inflammatory conditions such as rheumatoid arthritis, autoimmune conditions and so on.

Immunostimulants include:
    Bacterial vaccines
Colony stimulating factors
    Interferons
    Interleukin
    Immune globulins   *

Immunosuppressive agents include:
    Calcineurin inhibitors
    Interleukin inhibitors

Selective immunosuppressants such as
    TNF Alfa Inhibitors
Predisone
Glucocortisone.

Immunostimulants

Immunostimulants are substances that stimulate the immune system. Specific immunostimulants such as vaccines stimulate an immune response to specific antigenic types. Non-specific immunostimulants do not have antigenic specificity and are widely used in chronic infections, immunodeficiency, autoimmunity and neoplastic diseases.

In healthy individuals immune globulins are made by plasma cells when exposed by an immunogen such as a virus. Immune globulins act as antibodies against an infection. They are made up of different classes and subclasses of molecules. The immune globulin used for therapeutic purposes is made from healthy human blood that has a high level of antibodies. Immune globulins are given to those with a weak immune system to strengthen or act as the body's natural immune system. It decreases the risk of infection in the immunocompromised patients, who are unable to make antibodies themselves. *Hizentra* and *Gamunex* are commercially available injectables.

Bacterial Vaccines: Bacterial vaccines contain killed or attenuated bacteria that activate the immune system. Antibodies are built against that particular bacteria, and prevents bacterial infection later. An example of a bacterial vaccine is the Tuberculosis vaccine. *Prevnar* and *Pneumovax* are commercially available injectables.

Colony Stimulating Factors: Colony stimulating factors are glycoproteins that promote production of white blood cells (mainly granulocytes such as neutrophils), in response to infection. Administration of exogenous colony stimulating factors stimulates the stem cells in the bone marrow to produce more of the particular white blood cells. The new white blood cells migrate into the blood and fight the infection. Colony stimulating factors are used in patients who are undergoing cancer treatment that causes low white blood cell counts (neutropenia) and puts the patient at risk of infection. Colony stimulating factors tend to reduce the time where patients are neutropenic. One widely advertised injectable is pegfilgastim *(Neulasta)*.

Interferons: Interferons are proteins produced by host cells that are infected with viruses, bacteria and other unknown nucleic acids. Interferons also activate other cells that serve as part of the immune system and destroy invading pathogens. Interferons are classed as: alpha (from white cells), beta (from fibroblasts) and gamma (from lymphocytes). Interferons enhance the immune system in many ways so can be used to treat different conditions involving the immune system. Interferons used therapeutically are manufactured using recombinant DNA technology. Interferon alphas treat viral infections (chronic hepatitis, human papillomavirus) and cancer (hairy cell leukemia, AIDS related - Kaposi sarcoma, malignant melanoma).
Interferon betas are used to treat or slow down the progression of multiple sclerosis.
Interferon gamma is used to treat chronic granulomatous disease. *Avonex* and *Rebim* are widely available.

Interleukins: These are a group of cytokines which are synthesized by lymphocytes, monocytes, macrophages, and certain other cells. They function especially in regulation of the immune system. They are used to treat kidney cancer or skin cancer than has spread to other parts of the body, and help prevent low platelet counts caused by treatment with some cancer medicines. *Proleukin* and *Neumega* are widely available.

Therapeutic Vaccines: Therapeutic vaccines are vaccines which are intended to treat or cure a disorder or disease by stimulating the immune system. Therapeutic vaccines may be used to treat certain types of cancer, by stimulating the body's immune system to help it respond against certain cancer cells. *Provenge* (sipuleucel-T) is used for this purpose.

Viral Vaccines: Viral vaccines contain either inactivated viruses or attenuated (alive but not capable of causing disease) viruses. Inactivated or killed viral vaccines contain viruses, which have lost their ability to replicate and in order for it to bring about a response it contains more antigen than live vaccines. Attenuated or live vaccines contain the live form of the virus. These viruses are not pathogenic but are able to induce an immune response. The *Modena* and *Pfizer COVID-19* vaccines currently available are examples of these.

Immunosuppressants

Immunosuppressive agents are drugs that suppress the immune system and reduce the risk of rejection of foreign bodies such as transplant organs. Different classes of immunosuppressive agents have different mechanism of action. Now immunosuppressive agents are used as cancer chemotherapy, in autoimmune diseases such as rheumatoid arthritis and to treat severe allergy. As immunosuppressive agents lower the immunity there is increased risk of infection.

Types of immunosuppressive agent include:

      Calcineurin inhibitors

Interleukin inhibitors
Other immunosuppressants
Selective immunosuppressants
TNF alfa inhibitors

Calcineurin inhibitors: These are medicines which inhibit the action of calcineurin. Calcineurin is an enzyme that activates T-cells of the immune system. T-cells (also called T-lymphocytes) are a type of white blood cell that play a key role in cell-mediated immunity. Because calcineurin inhibitors suppress the immune system they are known as immunosuppressants. Topical calcineurin inhibitors (pimecrolimus, tacrolimus) may be used to treat inflammatory skin conditions such as atopic dermatitis when other treatments have failed. Oral and injectable calcineurin inhibitors (cyclosporine, tacrolimus) are used for both the induction and maintenance of postoperative immunosuppression after organ transplant surgery. *Neoral* (cyclosporine) is widely used.

Interleukin inhibitors: Interleukin inhibitors are immunosuppressive agents which inhibit the action of interleukins. Interleukins are a group of cytokines which are synthesized by lymphocytes, monocytes, macrophages, and certain other cells. They function especially in regulation of the immune system. They are used to treat moderate-to-severe inflammatory skin conditions that cannot be controlled with topical medicines. It is also used together with other medications to treat moderate-to-severe asthma that is not controlled with other asthma medicines in adults and children. *Dupixent* (dupilumab) is widely used.

Miscellaneous Immunosuppressants:

Immunosuppressive agents are drugs that suppress the immune system and reduce the risk of rejection of foreign bodies such as transplant organs. Different classes of immunosuppressive agents have different mechanism of action. Now immunosuppressive agents are used as cancer chemotherapy, in autoimmune diseases such as rheumatoid arthritis and to treat severe allergy. As immunosuppressive agents lower the immunity there is increased risk of infection. Immunosuppressants can be divided into classes including calcineurin inhibitors, interleukin inhibitors, selective immunosuppressants and TNF alfa inhibitors. Immunosuppressants that do not fit into these classes are categorized as other immunosuppressants. This category includes:

Azathioprine (*Azasan, Imuran*) - Kidney transplants; severe RA
Enalidomide (*Revlimid*) - multiple myeloma; myeolodysplastic anemia
Pomalidomide (*Pomalyst*) - multiple meloma; Kaposi's sarcoma
Methotrexate (*Otrexup, Rasuvo, Rheumatrex, Trexall*) - severe psoriasis; RA; polyarticular-course juvenile RA
Thalomid (thalidomide) - used together with dexamethasone to treat multiple myeloma and leprosy.

Selective Immunosuppressants:
These are drugs that suppress the immune system due to a selective point of action. They are used to reduce the risk of rejection in organ transplants, in autoimmune diseases and can be use as cancer chemotherapy. As immunosuppressive agents lower the immunity there is increased risk of infection. These include:

Xolair (omalizumab) - severe allergies; chronic urticaria; nasal polyps
Entyvio (vedolizumab) - severe ulcerative colitis and Crohn's disease
Tysabri (natalizumab) - MS, severe Crohn's disease
Gilenya (fingolimod) - MS
Tecfidera (dimethyl fumarate) - MS
Aubagio (teriflunomide) - MS
Orencia (abatacept) - severe RA; psoriatic arthritis
Benlysta (belimumab) - SLE
CellCept (mycophenolic acid) - kidney transplantation
Arava (leflunomide) - severe RA
Afinitor (everolimus) - kidney and liver transplantation
Raptiva (efalizumab) - plaque psoriasis in adults
Myfortic (mycophenolic acid) - kidney transplantation
Kesimpta (ofatumumab) - relapsing MS
Soliris (eculizumab) - paroxysmal nocturnal hemoglobinuria
Mayzent (siponimod) - secondary progressive MS
Zortress (everolimus) - kidney transplantation

TNF Alpha: TNF-alfa (alpha) inhibitors (TNF-alpha) are a group of medicines that suppress the body's natural response to tumor necrosis factor (TNF), a protein produced by white blood cells that is involved in early inflammatory events. TNF-alfa inhibitors treat a wide range of inflammatory conditions such as rheumatoid arthritis (RA), psoriatic arthritis, juvenile arthritis, Crohn's disease, ulcerative colitis, ankylosing spondylitis, and psoriasis. These include:

Adalimumab *(Amjevita, Hulio, Humira, Hyrimoz,)*
Etanercept *(Enbrel)*

Infliximab (*Remicade*)
Golimumab (*Simponi*)
Certolizumab (*Cimzia*)
Infliximab (*Inflectra, Ixifi, Renflexis*)

Prednisone: Prednisone is a glucocorticoid medication mostly used to suppress the immune system and decrease inflammation in conditions such as asthma, COPD, and rheumatologic diseases. It is also used to treat high blood calcium due to cancer and adrenal insufficiency along with other steroids. It is taken by mouth. Common side effects with long-term use include:

Cataracts
Bone loss
Easy bruising
Muscle weakness
Thrush oral candidiasis)
Weight gain
Edema
Hypertension
Increased risk of infection
Psychosis

It is generally considered safe in pregnancy and low doses appear to be safe when breastfeeding. After prolonged use, prednisone needs to be stopped very gradually, except in the case of Addison's disease (severe adrenal insufficiency) where the patient is kept on minimal doses replicating the quantity that would be produced in functioning Adrenal glands.
This mechanism leads to dependence in a short time and can be dangerous if medications are withdrawn too quickly. The body must have time to begin synthesis of

CRH and ACTH and for the adrenal glands to begin functioning normally again.

Fludrocortisone: Fludrocortisone is a steroid that helps reduce inflammation in the body. It is very often administered with Prednisone.
Fludrocortisone is used to treat conditions in which the body does not produce enough of its own steroids, such as Addison's disease. Users of Fludrocortisone need to avoid people who have infections: exposure to chickenpox or measles can be serious or fatal in patients who are using fludrocortisone.

One cannot receive a smallpox vaccine while using fludrocortisone and other vaccines should be subject to medical discretion while taking fludrocortisone. The more common side effects that can occur with fludrocortisone include:

Salt and water retention
 High blood pressure
 Muscle pain and weakness
 Headaches
 Glaucoma (increased pressure in your eyes)
 Feeling thirsty all the time

NEUROLOGICAL DRUGS

These include autonomic neurological and neuromuscular drugs (Alzheimers drugs, Antiseizure drugs, Movement disorder drugs, and Antiepiletpc/Antispasmodic drugs)

Within autonomic neuropharmacology, there are four specific categories of drugs based on how they affect the ANS:

Cholinomimetics/cholinesterase antagonists
Anticholinergics
Adrenoreceptor agonists/sympathomimetics
Adrenoreceptor antagonists

The clinical indications of medications from each of the four categories are listed below. Important to note is that this is not a complete list due to the vastness of drugs available; the drugs included are representative of each category.

Cholinomimetics/Cholinesterase Antagonists:

Cholinomimetics are a class of drugs that mimic the action of acetylcholine, a neurotransmitter involved in many functions including muscle activation, heart rate regulation, and brain function. These drugs can either directly stimulate acetylcholine receptors (direct-acting) or increase the availability of acetylcholine in the synaptic cleft (indirect-acting).

Bethanechol - postoperative and neurogenic ileus (colon/SI paralysis) and urinary retention (*Duvoid, Urecholine*)
     Pilocarpine - glaucoma and alleviating the symptoms of Sjogren's syndrome (an immune system disorder characterized by dry eyes and dry mouth) (*Salagen, Isoptocarpine*)
     Nicotine - found in smoking cessation regimens

Cholinesterase inhibitors (neostigmine, edrophonium, pyridostigmine, physostigmine):

These are used in the diagnosis and treatment of myasthenia gravis, maintenance treatment of Alzheimer disease, and specifically neostigmine used commonly with glycopyrrolate to reverse neuromuscular blockade in postoperative anesthesia practice. Cholinesterase inhibitors, also known as cholinesterase antagonists, work by preventing the breakdown of acetylcholine, thus enhancing cholinergic transmission. This class of drugs is used in various clinical settings.

Widely available drugs of this category are *Stimin, Prostimin* and *Bloxiverz*.

Anticholinergics:

Anticholinergics are a class of drugs that block the action of acetylcholine, a neurotransmitter involved in many functions in the body, including muscle contractions and various autonomic processes. By inhibiting acetylcholine, anticholinergics can help treat a range of conditions.

Atropine - used in ACLS guidelines to correct bradyarrhythmias and in ophthalmic surgery as a retinal dilator

Ipratropium and tiotropium - correct acute exacerbations of bronchospasm (asthma, COPD), as well as exacerbation prophylaxis for those conditions (*Spiriva*)

Scopolamine - prevents motion sickness and postoperative nausea/vomiting (*Transderm-Scop, Triscopo*)

Oxybutynin - urge incontinence and postoperative bladder spasm (*Oxytrol*)

Dicyclomine, glycopyrrolate - for reducing diarrhea in IBS; glycopyrrolate can also be added to cholinesterase reversal of neuromuscular blockades in postoperative anesthesia care to prevent bronchospasm and is currently in investigation as a treatment in COPD (*Cyclomin*)

Phenoxybenzamine, phentolamine - used to correct high catecholamine states (High levels of catecholamines* may indicate a wide variety of health conditions, including acute anxiety, severe stress, both cancerous and noncancerous tumors, and Menkes syndrome, a disorder that affects copper levels in the body) (*Dibenzyline*)

Prazosin, doxazosin, terazosin, tamsulosin - indicated to correct urinary retention in benign prostatic hyperplasia (*Minizide, Minipress*)

Catcholamines include adrenaline/epinephrine, norepinephrine and dopamine)

Adrenoreceptor agonists and sympathomimetics

These are classes of drugs that mimic the effects of the sympathetic nervous system, which is involved in the "fight or flight" response.

Adrenoreceptor agonists stimulate adrenoreceptors (also known as adrenergic receptors), which are activated by the neurotransmitters norepinephrine and epinephrine. These receptors are classified into alpha and beta subtypes:

Alpha-1 Agonists: These increase blood pressure by causing vasoconstriction. Examples include *phenylephrine* and *methoxamine*.

Alpha-2 Agonists: These reduce blood pressure and can have sedative effects by decreasing sympathetic outflow. Examples include *clonidine* and *dexmedetomidine*.

Beta-1 Agonists: These increase heart rate and contractility. An example is *dobutamine*.

Beta-2 Agonists: These relax bronchial smooth muscle and are used in the treatment of asthma and COPD. Examples include *albuterol* and *salbutamol*. Sympathomimetics are drugs that mimic the effects of sympathetic nervous system activation, generally by stimulating adrenoreceptors or increasing the release of norepinephrine and epinephrine. They can be classified based on their mechanism of action:

Direct-Acting Sympathomimetics: These drugs directly stimulate adrenoreceptors. Examples include:

Phenylephrine: A selective alpha-1 agonist used as a decongestant.
Albuterol: A beta-2 agonist used for bronchodilation in asthma.

Indirect-Acting Sympathomimetics: These increase the release of norepinephrine or inhibit its reuptake. Examples include:

Amphetamines: Increase norepinephrine release and are used to treat attention deficit hyperactivity disorder (ADHD) and narcolepsy.

Cocaine: Blocks the reuptake of norepinephrine and dopamine.

Both adrenoreceptor agonists and sympathomimetics can have various therapeutic uses, including the management of cardiovascular conditions, respiratory issues, and central nervous system disorders. They can also have side effects, such as increased heart rate, hypertension, and anxiety, depending on their specific actions and targets.

Adrenoreceptor Antagonists

Adrenoreceptor antagonists, also known as adrenergic blockers or adrenergic antagonists, are drugs that inhibit the action of neurotransmitters like norepinephrine and epinephrine (adrenaline) at adrenergic receptors. These receptors are classified into alpha and beta subtypes, and the antagonists are correspondingly classified based on the receptors they block:

Alpha-Adrenergic Antagonists (Alpha Blockers) block alpha-1 receptors, which are found primarily in blood vessels, leading to vasodilation and a reduction in blood pressure. They are used to treat conditions such as hypertension and benign prostatic hyperplasia (BPH). Examples include *Prazosin, Terazosin* and *Doxazosin*.

Alpha-2 Antagonists block alpha-2 receptors, which can increase the release of norepinephrine. They are less commonly used clinically but can be found in certain antidepressants. An example includes *Yohimbine*.

Beta-Adrenergic Antagonists (Beta Blockers) block both beta-1 and beta-2 receptors. They are used to manage conditions such as hypertension, angina, and arrhythmias, but are avoided in patients with asthma due to their effect on bronchoconstriction. Examples include *Propranolol* and *Nadolol.*

Selective Beta-1 Blockers (Cardioselective Beta Blockers) primarily block beta-1 receptors found in the heart, reducing heart rate and contractility. They are preferred in patients with respiratory conditions. Examples include *Atenolol, Metoprolol* and *Bisoprolol.*
Mixed Alpha and Beta Blockers block both alpha and beta receptors and are used in the management of hypertension and heart failure. Examples include *Labetalol* and *Carvedilol.*

Both alpha and beta blockers are used to lower blood pressure. Beta blockers are widely used for angina, arrhythmias, heart failure, and after myocardial infarction to reduce cardiac workload and oxygen demand. They are also used in Benign Prostatic Hyperplasia (BPH) as well as Migraine prevention and Glaucoma.

Anti-Seizure Medications

Anti-seizure medications (anticonvulsants) were originally designed to treat epilepsy, but are now also used to quiet the severe pain often caused by nerve damage. Anti-seizure medications appear to interfere with the overactive transmission of pain signals sent from damaged nerves (neuropathy) or overly sensitized nerves, as in fibromyalgia.

Some anti-seizure drugs work particularly well for certain conditions.

Carbamazepine (*Carbatrol, Tegretol*, others) is widely prescribed for trigeminal neuralgia, a condition that can cause searing facial pain that feels like an electric shock.

Gabapentin and *Pregabalin* are particularly effective in the treatment of postherpetic neuralgia, diabetic neuropathy and pain caused by a spinal cord injury.

These medications are removed from the body by the kidneys, so if kidney function is impaired, the dose may need to be adjusted. Anti-seizure drugs have been used to treat nerve pain for many years, but may require regular monitoring.

Depending on the type of pain, other anti-seizure drugs used may include:

>Carbamazepine (*Epitol*)
>Oxcarbazepine (*Trileptal, Oxtellar XR*)
>Lamotrigine (*Lamictal*)
>Phenytoin (*Dilantin*)
>Valproic acid (*Depakene*)

Alzheimers Drugs

Alzheimers is a progressive, neurodegenerative disease characterised by loss of function and death of nerve cells in several areas of the brain leading to loss of cognitive function such as memory and language. The cause of nerve cell death is unknown but the cells are recognised by the appearance of unusual helical protein filaments in the nerve cells. The drugs listed for its treatment do not cure Alzheimers disease, but may slow and lessen the progression of symptoms.

The Food and Drug Administration (FDA) has approved two types of drugs specifically to treat symptoms of Alzheimer's disease.

* Cholinesterase inhibitors
* Memantine

There are a large number of recently introduced drugs that are used to treat Alzheimers, but the most widely prescribed is the cholinesterase-inhibitors

Donepizil (*Aricept*)
Galantamine (*Razadyne*)
Rivastigminbev (*Exelon*)

Donepezil: Sold under the brand name *Aricept*, this medication is a cholinesterase (AChE) inhibitor prescribed to help those diagnosed with mild, moderate, and severe Alzheimer's disease. Donepezil is taken as a pill, or dissolving tablet for those unable to swallow, with side effects that commonly include gastrointestinal issues and sleep disruption. First approved by the FDA in 1996, this drug was classified to treat all stages of Alzheimer's in 2006 after extensive clinical trials showing its potential to delay the onset of memory loss and cognitive abilities. It is approved to treat all stages of the disease. It's taken once a day as a pill.

Galantamine: This medication is sold under the name *Razadyne*, and it is a cholinesterase inhibitor that is effective and mild to moderate Alzheimer's disease. According to the NIH, the main differences between this medication and donepezil are that galantamine users' caregivers recorded less "burdens" during their patients' time on the medication, in a 2003 clinical trial. Both medications have similar amounts of side effects, but galantamine users experience a skin rash sometimes, in addition to the standard intestinal issues caused by the tendency of cholinesterase inhibitors to increase stomach acid production. It is approved to treat mild to moderate Alzheimer's. It's taken as a pill once a day or as an extended-release capsule twice a day.

Rivastigmine: This medication, also known as *Exelon*, is used to improve memory and cognition in those diagnosed with mild to severe Alzheimer's disease. As in other cholinesterase inhibitors, this medication is helpful in treating dementia-related memory loss, but not in the case of frontotemporal dementia (FTD). It is approved to treat mild to moderate Alzheimer's. It's taken as a pill once a day or as an extended-release capsule twice a day.

Memantine: Sold under the name *Namenda*, this is approved by the FDA for treatment of moderate to severe Alzheimer's disease. It works by regulating the activity of glutamate, a messenger chemical widely involved in brain functions, including learning and memory. It's taken as a pill or syrup. Common side effects include dizziness, headache, confusion and agitation. The FDA has also approved a combination of donepezil and memantine (*Namzaric*), which is taken as a capsule. Side effects include headache, dizziness, nausea and diarrhea.

GASTROINTESTINAL DRUGS

Gastrointestinal (GI) agents include many different classes of drugs that are used to treat gastrointestinal disorders.

They can be classed as:

> Antacids (incl. Proton Pump Inhibitors)
> Antidiarrheals,
> Promotility agents
> Digestive enzymes
> Functional bowel disorder agents
> Gallstone solubilizing agents
> 5-Aminosalicylates,

Antacids:

An antacid is a substance which neutralizes stomach acidity and is used to relieve heartburn, indigestion or an upset stomach. Some antacids have been used in the treatment of constipation and diarrhea. Currently marketed antacids contain salts of aluminum, calcium, magnesium, or sodium. Some preparations contain a combination of two salts, such as magnesium carbonate and aluminum hydroxide. Antacids are linked to an increased risk of gastrointestinal infections.

Proton Pump Inhibitors (PPIs) are medications that cause a profound prolonged reduction of stomach acid production. They do so by inhibiting the stomach's $H+/K+$ATPase proton pump, and are the most potent inhibitors of acid secretion available. Proton pump inhibitors such as *Prilosec* (omeprazole) and *Nexium* (esomeprazole) are among the most widely prescribed medications in the world. Used for the treatment of gastroesophageal reflux disease (GERD), they are effective and relatively safe when used on a short-term basis. Common adverse effects include headache, nausea, diarrhea, abdominal pain, fatigue, and dizziness.

H2 Antagonists: These block histamine-induced gastric acid secretion from the parietal cells of the gastric mucosa (lining of the stomach). H2 antagonists are used to treat gastroesophageal reflux disease (GERD), gastrointestinal ulcers and other gastrointestinal hypersecretory conditions. They are used in the prevention and treatment of duodenal ulcer, erosive esophagitis, helicobacter pylori infections, peptic ulcer, and upper GI tract hemorrhages. Side effects may include dizziness, fainting, fast or pounding heartbeat, continuing or severe headache, lightheadedness, and nervousness.

Widely used H2 antagonists include:

> Famotidine (*Zantac*)
> Famotidine (Pepcid)
> Nizatidine (*Axid*)
> Cimetidine (*Taxid*)

Anti-Diarrheal Drugs

These include both prescription and non-prescription drugs:

Prescription drugs include:

Loperamide (*Imodium*):
Reduces bowel movements by slowing the rhythm of digestion and is often prescribed for chronic diarrhea, including diarrhea caused by inflammatory bowel disease.

Diphenoxylate and Atropine (*Lomotil*):
Slows bowel movements.and is used for the treatment of acute and chronic diarrhea.

Eluxadoline (*Viberzi*):
Acts on opioid receptors in the gut to reduce bowel contractions. Is used specifically for diarrhea-predominant irritable bowel syndrome (IBS-D).

Rifaximin *(Xifaxan): An antibiotic that reduces or alters gut bacteria. Often used for travelers' diarrhea and IBS.*

Alosetron (*Lotronex*): Blocks serotonin signals that can trigger bowel movement and pain.
Ordinarily reserved for severe IBS in women that hasn't responded to other treatments.

Over-the-Counter Drug Include:

Loperamide (*Imodium A-D*): This is the same as prescription loperamide at a higher potency, and reduces bowel movements. It is f*or short-term relief of acute diarrhea.*

Bismuth Subsalicylate *(Pepto-Bismol, Kaopectate):* These coat the stomach lining and have antimicrobial properties. These treat diarrhea, nausea, and upset stomach.

Kaolin and Pectin: These absorb bacteria and toxins in the gut, reduces bowel movements and are traditionally used for mild to moderate diarrhea

Promotility Agents

Drugs used in the management of intestinal motility disorders include:

Cholinergic agonists
Prokinetic agents
Opioid antagonists

The agents that are most useful in the treatment of these disorders include Neostigmine, Bethanechol, Metoclopramide, Cisapride, and Loperamide. Neostigmine appears to increase antral and intestinal motor activity in patients with hypomotility, including intestinal dysmotility.

Cholinergic Agonists: Excessive parasympathetic suppression appears to be involved in the genesis of intestinal pseudo-obstruction. Cholinergic agents may allow early resolution of pseudo-obstruction and obviate surgery.

An example of one such drug is *Bethanechol* (Urecholine)

Prokinetic Agents: Prokinetics are promotility agents, proposed for use with severe constipation-predominant symptoms.

Examples of these include:

Metoproclamide (*Reglan, Metozolv*)
Cisapride (*Propulsid*)
Tegaserod (*Zelnorm*)

Tegaserod is used to treat irritable bowel syndrome with constipation (IBS-C) or chronic idiopathic constipation

(CIC) in women younger than 55 years who meet specific guidelines who have no known or preexisting heart disease. Tegaserod is used for short-term treatment of women with IBS in which constipation is the predominant symptom. It is also indicated to treat CIC.

Opioid Antagonists

Peripherally selective opioid antagonists are used to treat constipation in patients who have advanced illness requiring chronic opioid analgesia and are unresponsive to laxatives.

Examples of these include:

Naloxegol (*Movantik*)
Methylnaltrexone (*Relistor*)

Methylnaltrexone is a peripherally acting mu-opioid receptor antagonist. It selectively displaces opioids from mu-opioid receptors outside the central nervous system (CNS), including those located in the GI tract, thereby decreasing constipating effects. Methylnaltrexone is indicated for opioid-induced constipation in patients with advanced illness who are receiving palliative care and whose response to laxatives has not been sufficient. It is a subcutaneous injection.

Digestive Enzymes

Prescription digestive enzymes are used to help individuals who have conditions that impair the production of natural digestive enzymes, such as chronic pancreatitis, cystic fibrosis, or pancreatic cancer. These enzymes assist in breaking down fats, proteins, and carbohydrates to aid in proper digestion and play a crucial role in managing conditions that affect the pancreas and overall digestion, helping patients maintain a better quality of life by improving nutrient absorption and reducing gastrointestinal symptoms. Gastrointestinal discomfort and allergic reactions are occasional side effects..

Here are some commonly utilized digestive enzymes:

Pancrelipase (*Creon, Pancreaze, Zenpep, Viokace*): Contains a mix of lipase, protease, and amylase derived from pig pancreas. Used to treat pancreatic enzyme insufficiency due to conditions like cystic fibrosis, chronic pancreatitis, or after pancreatic surgery.

Pancreatin: Similar to pancrelipase, it contains a mixture of digestive enzymes (lipase, protease, and amylase). Treats enzyme insufficiency due to chronic pancreatitis or cystic fibrosis.

Lactase *(Lactaid)*: Contains the enzyme lactase. Used for individuals with lactose intolerance to help digest lactose found in dairy products.

Alpha-Galactosidase *(Beano)*: Contains the enzyme alpha-galactosidase. Helps break down complex carbohydrates found in legumes and certain vegetables to reduce gas and bloating.

Lipase: Contains the enzyme lipase. Prescribed for individuals with fat malabsorption issues, often in combination with other enzymes.

Drugs for Functional Bowel Disorders

Drugs for Functional bowel disorders (such as Irritable Bowel Syndrome (IBS) and Functional Dyspepsia) often require a multifaceted treatment approach. Prescription drugs used to manage these conditions focus on alleviating symptoms such as pain, constipation, and diarrhea. These prescription medications can help manage the complex and often fluctuating symptoms of functional bowel disorders, improving the quality of life for many patients.
This category of drug includes antispasmodics, fiber supplements, laxatives, antidiarrheals, serotonin modulators, and anti-depressants.

Here are some commonly prescribed drugs for functional bowel disorders:

Antispasmodics:

Hyoscyamine (*Levsin, Anaspaz*): Reduces bowel spasms. Alleviates cramping and abdominal pain associated with IBS.

Dicyclomine (*Bentyl*): Relieves muscle spasms in the gastrointestinal tract. Used to treat IBS symptoms.

Fiber Supplements:

Psyllium (*Metamucil*): Adds bulk to stool and helps with both constipation and diarrhea. Often recommended for IBS to regulate bowel movements.

Laxatives:

Lubiprostone (*Amitiza*): Increases fluid secretion in the intestine to ease stool passage. Prescribed for IBS with constipation (IBS-C) and chronic idiopathic constipation.
Linaclotide (*Linzess*): Increases fluid in the intestines and speeds up movement. Treats IBS-and chronic idiopathic constipation.

Serotonin Modulators:
Alosetron (Lotronex): Blocks serotonin signals that can trigger bowel movement and pain. Reserved for severe IBS-D in women who haven't responded to other treatments.
Tegaserod (*Zelnorm*): Stimulates serotonin receptors to increase motility and fluid secretion in the gut. Used for IBS in women under 65.

Gallstone Solubilizing Agents

Prescription drugs used to dissolve gallstones are typically employed in cases where surgery is not an option or is undesirable. These medications are usually most effective on cholesterol gallstones and less effective on pigment stones. These medications can take months or even years to fully dissolve gallstones, and they are not always successful. Regular monitoring through ultrasound or other imaging techniques is necessary to track progress. These drugs are generally effective only on small, cholesterol-rich gallstones and are less effective on larger or calcified stones.

Ursodiol and chenodiol are the primary prescription medications used to dissolve cholesterol gallstones and offer a non-surgical option for certain patients, though they require a long-term commitment and regular medical supervision to ensure effectiveness and manage side effects.

Here are the commonly prescribed gallstone solubilizing drugs:

Ursodiol (*Actigall, Urso*): Ursodeoxycholic acid is a bile acid that reduces the cholesterol content of bile, thereby dissolving cholesterol gallstones. Used to dissolve small, non-calcified cholesterol gallstones and to prevent gallstone formation in obese patients experiencing rapid weight loss.

Chenodiol (*Chenix*): Chenodeoxycholic acid works by decreasing the production of cholesterol in the liver and reducing the amount of cholesterol in bile, which helps dissolve cholesterol gallstones. Primarily used for the non-surgical treatment of radiolucent cholesterol gallstones.

5-Aminosalicylates

5-Aminosalicylates (5-ASAs) are a class of drugs primarily used to treat inflammatory bowel diseases (IBD) such as ulcerative colitis and, to a lesser extent, Crohn's disease. These medications work by reducing inflammation in the lining of the intestines.

These 5-ASA drugs play a key role in managing inflammatory bowel diseases, helping to reduce inflammation and maintain remission, thereby improving the quality of life for many patients.

Here are some commonly prescribed 5-ASA drugs, which are administered orally or by rectal suppository:

Mesalamine / Mesalazine: (*Asacol HD, Pentasa, Lialda, Apriso, Delzicol, Rowasa, Canasa*) Acts locally in the colon to reduce inflammation by inhibiting the production of inflammatory chemicals (prostaglandins and leukotrienes). Treats mild to moderate ulcerative colitis and helps maintain remission.

-

Sulfasalazine: (*Azulfidine, Azulfidine EN-tabs*) Combination of sulfapyridine and mesalamine. Sulfapyridine helps deliver mesalamine to the colon where it exerts its anti-inflammatory effects. Used for the treatment of ulcerative colitis (and also for rheumatoid arthritis.)

Olsalazine: (*Dipentum*) Two mesalamine molecules linked together, which are split in the colon to release active mesalamine. Used as a maintenance therapy for ulcerative colitis.

Balsalazide: (*Colazal, Giazo*), A prodrug that is converted into mesalamine in the colon to exert anti-inflammatory effects. Treats mild to moderate ulcerative colitis.

ANTI-INFLAMMATORY MEDICATIONS

Anti-inflammatory medications are a crucial part of drug therapy for alternative health practitioners. Many of these are discussed in detail under "Analgesics" above.

These medications work by reducing inflammation in the body, which can help alleviate pain, swelling, and stiffness associated with various health conditions. It is important for practitioners to understand the different types of anti-inflammatory medications available and how they can be used to effectively treat their patients.

Nonsteroidal Anti-Inflammatory Drugs (NSAIDS):

Nonsteroidal anti-inflammatory drugs (NSAIDs) are commonly used to reduce inflammation and pain and have already been discussed. These medications work by blocking the production of prostaglandins, which are chemicals in the body that cause inflammation. NSAIDs can be used to treat a variety of conditions, including arthritis, muscle strains, and menstrual cramps.

It is important for practitioners to be aware of the potential side effects of NSAIDs, such as stomach ulcers and kidney damage, and to monitor their patients closely while they are taking these medications.

These include Ibuprofen, Naproxen Aspirin and Meloxicam and Diclofenac.

Corticosteroids:

Corticosteroids, which have been discussed above in detail, are another type of anti-inflammatory medication that can be used to reduce inflammation in the body.

These medications work by suppressing the immune system, which can help reduce inflammation and pain. Corticosteroids are often used to treat conditions such as asthma, rheumatoid arthritis, and inflammatory bowel disease.

Practitioners should be aware of the potential side effects of corticosteroids, such as weight gain, high blood pressure, and an increased risk of infection, and should closely monitor their patients while they are taking these medications.

Disease-Modifying Antirheumatic Drugs (DMARDs):

Another type of anti-inflammatory medication that practitioners may encounter is disease-modifying antirheumatic drugs (DMARDs). These medications are often used to treat autoimmune conditions, such as rheumatoid arthritis, by suppressing the immune system and reducing inflammation. DMARDs can help slow the progression of these conditions and improve the quality of life for patients.

Practitioners should be aware of the potential side effects of DMARDs, such as liver damage and an increased risk of infection and should closely monitor their patients while they are taking these medications.

These medications are prescribed based on the severity and specific characteristics of the disease, as well as the patient's response to treatment.

The most commonly prescribed anti-inflammatory Disease-Modifying Anti-Rheumatic Drugs (DMARDs) include:

Methotrexate: Often the first-line treatment for rheumatoid arthritis and other inflammatory conditions. It works by

inhibiting the metabolism of folic acid, which reduces the proliferation of immune cells (*Trexall, Rheumatrex*)
Sulfasalazine: Used to treat rheumatoid arthritis and inflammatory bowel disease. It reduces inflammation by suppressing the immune system (*Azulfdine*)
      Leflunomide: This drug inhibits the synthesis of pyrimidine, leading to a decrease in lymphocyte proliferation and reduction of inflammation (*Arava*)
Hydroxychloroquine: Originally used to treat malaria, it is now commonly prescribed for rheumatoid arthritis and lupus. It modulates the immune system and has anti-inflammatory properties (*Plauenil*)
Azathioprine: An immunosuppressant that is used to treat rheumatoid arthritis and other autoimmune conditions by inhibiting the proliferation of immune cells (*Imuran*)
Cyclosporine: This immunosuppressant is used for rheumatoid arthritis and other autoimmune diseases. It inhibits the activity of T cells, reducing inflammation. (*Neoral, Sandimmune*)
Biologic DMARDs: These are newer agents that target specific components of the immune system. Common biologics include:
TNF inhibitors: Examples are Adalimumab (*Humira*), Etanercept (*Enbrel*), and Infliximab (*Remicade*).
IL-6 inhibitors: Such as Tocilizumab (*Actemra*).
B-cell inhibitors: Like Rituximab (*Rituxan*).
      T-cell inhibitors: Such as Abatacept (*Orencia*).

Overall, anti-inflammatory medications are an important part of drug therapy for alternative health practitioners. These medications can help reduce inflammation and pain in patients with a variety of conditions, improving their quality of life. Practitioners should be familiar with the different types of anti-inflammatory medications available, their mechanisms of action, and potential side effects. By using these medications judiciously and monitoring their patients closely, practitioners can effectively treat inflammation and help their patients achieve better health outcomes.

ANTIHISTAMINES

Antihistamines are a class of pharmaceutical drugs commonly used to treat allergic reactions and symptoms related to allergies. These medications work by blocking the effects of histamine, a compound produced by the body in response to allergens. Alternative health practitioners may find antihistamines to be a valuable tool in managing allergic conditions and providing relief to their patients.

Antihistamines can be used to alleviate a variety of allergy symptoms, including sneezing, itching, hives, and nasal congestion. They are also commonly used to treat symptoms of hay fever, allergic rhinitis, and allergic skin conditions. Alternative health practitioners should be aware of the potential side effects of antihistamines, which may include drowsiness, dry mouth, dizziness, and blurred vision.

Antihistamines are a valuable tool for alternative health practitioners in managing allergy symptoms and providing relief to their patients. By understanding the different types of antihistamines, their uses, and potential side effects, alternative health practitioners can make informed decisions when recommending these medications. It is important for practitioners to educate their patients about the proper use of antihistamines and consider non-pharmacological approaches to managing allergies.

It is important for alternative health practitioners to educate their patients about the proper use of antihistamines, including dosage instructions and potential drug-herb interactions. Patients should be advised to avoid driving or operating heavy machinery while taking antihistamines, especially those that cause drowsiness. Alternative health practitioners may also recommend non-pharmacological approaches to managing allergies, such as avoiding allergens and using natural remedies.

There are several types of antihistamines: first-generation and second-generation. Alternative health practitioners should consider these differences when discussing antihistamines with their patients. All work by blocking the action of histamine, a substance in the body that causes allergic symptoms. Antihistamines can be classified into several types based on their chemical structure and generation. Here are the main types:

First-Generation Antihistamines

These were the first antihistamines developed and tend to cause more drowsiness because they can cross the blood-brain barrier. Common first-generation antihistamines include:

Diphenhydramine (*Benadryl*)
Chlorpheniramine (*Chlor-Trimeton*)
Brompheniramine (*Dimetane*)
Clemastine (*Tavist*)

Hydroxyzine (*Atarax, Vistaril*)
Promethazine (*Phenergan*)

Second-Generation Antihistamines

These are newer antihistamines that are less likely to cause drowsiness because they are less likely to cross the blood-brain barrier. Common second-generation antihistamines include:

Loratadine (*Claritin*)
Cetirizine (*Zyrtec*)
Fexofenadine (*Allegra*)
Desloratadine (*Clarinex*)
Levocetirizine (*Xyzal*)

Third-Generation Antihistamines

These are derivatives of second-generation antihistamines designed to improve efficacy and reduce side effects. They are also less likely to cause drowsiness. Common third-generation antihistamines include:

Fexofenadine (*Allegra*)
Levocetirizine (*Xyzal*)
Desloratadine (*Clarinex*)

H2-Receptor Antagonists (H2 Blockers)

Although primarily used to reduce stomach acid production, H2 blockers also have antihistamine effects. They are often used for conditions like peptic ulcers and gastroesophageal reflux disease (GERD). Common H2 blockers include:

- Ranitidine (*Zantac*)
Famotidine (*Pepcid*)
Cimetidine (*Tagamet*)
Nizatidine (*Axid*)

Intranasal Antihistamines

These are administered through the nose and are used to treat nasal allergy symptoms. Common intranasal antihistamines include:

Azelastine (*Astelin, Astepro*)
Olopatadine (*Patanase*)
Fluticasone (*Flornase*) *Steroid

Ophthalmic Antihistamines

These are eye drops used to treat allergic conjunctivitis (eye allergies). Common ophthalmic antihistamines include:

Ketotifen (*Zaditor, Alaway*)
Olopatadine (*Patanol, Pataday*)
Azelastine (*Optivar*)

Each type of antihistamine has its own advantages and potential side effects, and the choice of which one to use depends on the specific symptoms and individual patient factors.

CHEMOTHERAPEUTIC AGENTS

Chemotherapeutic agents are an essential component of modern medicine, particularly in the treatment of cancer. These drugs work by targeting and destroying cancer cells, either by stopping their growth or by causing them to die. While the side effects of chemotherapy can be severe, they are often necessary to effectively combat the disease.

One of the challenges of using chemotherapeutic agents is that they can also harm healthy cells in the body, leading to a range of side effects. These can include nausea, fatigue, hair loss, and an increased risk of infection. Alternative health practitioners should be aware of these potential side effects and work closely with their patients to manage them effectively.

In recent years, there has been growing interest in the use of natural and alternative therapies to complement traditional chemotherapy. Some studies have suggested that certain herbs, supplements, and lifestyle changes can help to support the body's natural defenses and reduce the side effects of chemotherapy. Alternative health practitioners should stay informed about the latest research in this area and be prepared to discuss these options with their patients.

Ultimately, the use of chemotherapeutic agents is a complex and multifaceted aspect of modern medicine. Alternative health practitioners should approach the use of these drugs with caution and respect for their potential risks and benefits. By staying informed and working closely with their patients, they can help to ensure the best possible outcomes for those undergoing chemotherapy.

There are several different classes of chemotherapeutic agents, each with its own unique mechanism of action. Chemotherapy drugs are classified into several categories based on their chemical structure, mechanism of action, and the phase of the cell cycle they target. Here are the main categories. These include ankylating agents, antimetabolites, plant alkaloids, antitumor antibiotics, topoisomerase inhibitors, mitotic inhibitors, corticosteroids, miscellaneous antineoplastic agents, targeted therapy agents, hormones, and immunotherapy agents.

Alkylating Agents

Mechanism: These drugs work by adding an alkyl group to the DNA, which interferes with DNA replication and RNA transcription.
Examples: *Cyclophosphamide, Ifosfamide, Melphalan, Chlorambucil.*

Antimetabolites

Mechanism: These drugs mimic the building blocks of DNA and RNA, thereby interfering with DNA and RNA synthesis.
Examples: *Methotrexate, 5-Fluorouracil (5-FU), Cytarabine, Gemcitabine.*

Plant Alkaloids

Subcategories:

Vinca Alkaloids:
   Inhibit microtubule formation in mitotic spindle.
Examples: *Vincristine, Vinblastine, Vinorelbine.*

Taxanes: Stabilize microtubules and inhibit cell division.
Examples: *Paclitaxel, Docetaxel.*

Podophyllotoxins: Inhibit DNA topoisomerase II.
Examples: *Etoposide, Teniposide*.

Camptothecins: Inhibit DNA topoisomerase I.
Examples: Irinotecan, *Topotecan*.

Antitumor Antibiotics

Mechanism: These drugs bind to DNA and inhibit RNA synthesis or interfere with enzymes involved in DNA replication.
- Examples: *Doxorubicin, Daunorubicin, Bleomycin, Mitomycin C.*
-

Topoisomerase Inhibitors

Mechanism: These drugs inhibit the action of topoisomerase enzymes, which help unwind DNA for replication.
- Examples: *Irinotecan (Topoisomerase I inhibitor), Etoposide (Topoisomerase II inhibitor)*.

Mitotic Inhibitors

Mechanism: These drugs inhibit mitosis (cell division) by interfering with microtubules.
- Examples: *Paclitaxel, Docetaxel, Vincristine, Vinblastine*.

Corticosteroids

Mechanism: These are hormones that can kill cancer cells directly or reduce inflammation around tumors.
- Examples: *Prednisone, Dexamethasone*.

Miscellaneous Antineoplastic Agents
Mechanism: These drugs have unique mechanisms of action that do not fit neatly into other categories.
- Examples: *Asparaginase, Hydroxyurea, Mitotane*.

Targeted Therapies

Mechanism: These drugs target specific molecules involved in cancer cell growth and survival.
- Examples: *Imatinib, Trastuzumab, Erlotinib*.

Hormone Therapy

Mechanism: These drugs interfere with hormone production or hormone action to slow or stop the growth of hormone-sensitive tumors.
- Examples: *Tamoxifen, Anastrozole, Leuprolide*

Immunotherapy

Mechanism: These drugs enhance the body's immune system to fight cancer cells.
Examples: Pembrolizumab *(Keytruda),* Nivolumab (*Opdivo*), Ipilimumab (*Yervoy*)

TOPICAL MEDICATIONS

Topical medications are pharmaceutical drugs that are applied directly to the skin to treat various conditions and ailments. These medications come in the form of creams, ointments, gels, sprays, and patches, and are absorbed through the skin to target specific areas of the body. Alternative health practitioners often use topical medications as part of their treatment plans to provide relief from pain, inflammation, infections, and other skin-related issues.

One of the key benefits of using topical medications is that they can deliver medication directly to the affected area, allowing for faster and more targeted relief. This is especially useful for conditions such as arthritis, muscle strains, and skin infections, where localized treatment is necessary. Additionally, topical medications are generally well-tolerated and have fewer systemic side effects compared to oral medications, making them a safe and effective option for many patients.

There are several different types of topical medications available, each with its own unique properties and applications. For example, corticosteroid creams are commonly used to reduce inflammation and itching associated with conditions such as eczema and psoriasis, while antibiotic ointments are used to treat bacterial infections on the skin. Topical analgesics, such as lidocaine patches, are also popular for providing pain relief without the need for oral medications.

When dealing with or recommending topical medications, alternative health practitioners must consider several factors, including the patient's medical history, skin type, and potential drug interactions. It is important to educate patients on how to properly apply and use the medication to ensure maximum effectiveness and minimize the risk of side effects. Alternative health practitioners should also monitor patients closely for any signs of allergic reactions or adverse effects while using topical medications.

Overall, topical medications are a valuable tool in the arsenal of alternative health practitioners for treating a wide range of conditions. By understanding the different types of topical medications available and how to use them effectively, practitioners can provide their patients with safe and effective relief from pain, inflammation, and other skin-related issues. With proper education and monitoring, topical medications can be a valuable addition to any alternative health practitioner's treatment plan.

Topical medicines come in various forms and are used to treat a wide range of conditions. The most common types follow.

Skin Treatments

Topical Antibiotics
Used in treating bacterial infections of the skin, such as impetigo.
Mupirocin, Neomycin, Bacitracin

Topical Antifungals
Used in Treating fungal infections like athlete's foot, ringworm, and yeast infections.
Clotrimazole, Ketoconazole, Terbinafine

Topical Antiseptics
Used for cleaning wounds and preventing infection.

- Chlorhexidine, Povidone-iodine

Topical Corticosteroids
Reduces inflammation and itching in conditions like eczema, psoriasis, and dermatitis.
Hydrocortisone, Triamcinolone, Betamethasone
-

Topical Antivirals
Treats viral infections like herpes simplex (cold sores)
- Acyclovir, Penciclovir

Topical Retinoids
Treat acne, reducing wrinkles, and other skin conditions.
- Tretinoin, Adapalene, Tazarotene

Topical Immunomodulators
Used to treat inflammatory skin conditions like eczema when other treatments are not suitable.
- Tacrolimus, Pimecrolimus

Topical Anti-Inflammatories
Reduces inflammation and pain in conditions like arthritis.
Diclofenac, Ibuprofen

Topical Anti-Psoriatics
Treats psoriasis by reducing scaling and slowing skin cell growth.
Calcipotriene, Coal Tar

Topical Emollients and Moisturizers
Hydrates and protects skin, often used for dry skin conditions.
Urea, Lanolin
-

Topical Acne Treatments
Used in treating acne by reducing bacteria and inflammation.
- Benzoyl Peroxide, Clindamycin

Topical Rosacea Treatments
Treats rosacea by reducing redness and inflammation.
- Metronidazole, Azelaic Acid

Topical Anti-Pruritics
Uses: Relieving itching from various skin conditions.
- Pramoxine, Doxepin
-

Topical Hair Growth Stimulants
Promotes hair growth in conditions like androgenetic alopecia.
- Minoxidil

Topical Pain Relievers

Relieves pain from conditions like neuropathy and musculoskeletal pain.
- Lidocaine, Capsaicin

Ophthalmic Medications

Antibiotics: Ciprofloxacin, Erythromycin (for bacterial eye infections)
Antivirals: Trifluridine (for viral eye infections like herpes simplex)
Anti-inflammatories: Prednisolone, Dexamethasone (for inflammation)
Antihistamines: Ketotifen (for allergic conjunctivitis)

Glaucoma Medications: Latanoprost, Timolol (for reducing intraocular pressure)

Otic (Ear) Medications

Antibiotics: Ofloxacin, Neomycin (for bacterial ear infections)
Antifungals: Clotrimazole (for fungal ear infections)
Anti-inflammatories: Hydrocortisone (for reducing inflammation and itching)
Cerumenolytics: Carbamide Peroxide (for softening and removing earwax)

Topical Nasal Medications

Decongestants: Oxymetazoline, Phenylephrine (for reducing nasal congestion)
Corticosteroids: Fluticasone, Mometasone (for reducing inflammation in allergic rhinitis)
Anticholinergics: Ipratropium (for reducing nasal secretions)

Topical (Mouth)Oral Medications

Analgesics: Benzocaine, Lidocaine (for pain relief in oral sores and dental procedures)
Antifungals: Nystatin, Clotrimazole (for oral thrush)
Anti-inflammatories: Triamcinolone dental paste (for reducing inflammation in mouth ulcers)

Vaginal Medications

Antifungals: Clotrimazole, Miconazole (for yeast infections)
Antibacterials: Metronidazole (for bacterial vaginosis)

Hormonal Treatments: Estradiol cream (for vaginal atrophy and dryness)

Topical Rectal Medications

Anti-hemorrhoidal: Hydrocortisone, Witch Hazel (for treating hemorrhoids and rectal inflammation)
Local Anesthetics: Lidocaine (for pain relief in rectal conditions)

Topical Musculoskeletal Medications

Anti-inflammatories: Diclofenac gel (for arthritis and musculoskeletal pain)
Analgesics: Capsaicin cream (for neuropathic pain)

Topical Medications for Tobacco Addiction

Transdermal patches that release nicotine slowly over a period of time. They are applied to the skin and are available in various strengths to help people gradually reduce their nicotine
intake. Varieties commercially available include *NicoDerm CQ, Habitrol, Nicotinell* and *Nicotrol*.

REPRODUCTION MANAGEMENT DRUGS

Birth Control Drugs – Female

Hormonal Methods

Hormonal birth control for women includes a range of options designed to prevent ovulation, alter cervical mucus, or affect the uterine lining. Combined oral contraceptives (COCs) contain both estrogen and progestin and are the most commonly prescribed form.

These include brand-name drugs like Yasmin, Ortho Tri-Cyclen, and Alesse. Progestin-only pills (POPs), such as Micronor and Camila, are suitable for those who cannot take estrogen. Long-acting reversible contraceptives (LARCs) include hormonal intrauterine devices like Mirena and Skyla, as well as injectable depot medroxyprogesterone acetate (Depo-Provera) and subdermal implants like Nexplanon. Emergency contraceptives, such as Plan B (levonorgestrel) and Ella (ulipristal acetate), provide post-coital hormonal intervention. Transdermal patches like Xulane and vaginal rings like NuvaRing also fall under hormonal methods.

Non-Hormonal Methods

Non-hormonal birth control options for women include copper intrauterine devices such as Paragard, which act primarily by creating an inflammatory reaction in the uterus toxic to sperm. Barrier methods like diaphragms, cervical caps, and female condoms fall into this category, as do spermicidal gels like nonoxynol-9. Male birth control options remain limited and primarily involve barrier methods such as condoms and the permanent option of vasectomy. However, research into male hormonal contraceptives such as testosterone-progestin combinations or compounds like DMAU (dimethandrolone undecanoate) is ongoing.

Herbal Interactions

Several Ayurvedic herbs are known to interact with hormonal birth control methods, either by altering hormone metabolism, affecting liver enzyme pathways, or changing uterine and cervical physiology.

Ashoka (Saraca asoca) and Lodhra (Symplocos racemosa), used in regulating menstruation and fertility, may theoretically interfere with hormonal balance and modify uterine receptivity. Shatavari (Asparagus racemosus), a reproductive tonic, can modulate estrogenic activity and may potentiate or compete with exogenous hormones in oral contraceptives.

Similarly, herbs such as Guggulu (Commiphora mukul), known to stimulate liver enzymes like CYP3A4, affect the metabolism of synthetic estrogens and progestins, reducing their effectiveness. Triphala and turmeric, both widely used, also enhance liver detoxification pathways and reduce hormone levels by speeding clearance.

Birth Control Drugs – Male

Hormonal Methods

Male contraceptive drugs are currently under active development, though few options have reached widespread use or approval. They can be categorized into hormonal, non-hormonal, and mechanical methods. Hormonal male contraceptives involve suppressing production of testosterone and other gonadotropins such as luteinizing hormone (LH) and follicle-stimulating hormone (FSH). This leads to a reversible reduction in sperm production.

These combine synthetic progestins with testosterone or

its analogs to maintain libido and secondary sexual characteristics while inhibiting spermatogenesis. Examples under investigation include testosterone undecanoate injections, norethisterone enanthate, and gels like Nestorone combined with testosterone. These approaches may have side effects such as acne, mood swings, and changes in libido, similar to those seen in female hormonal contraceptives.

Non-Hormonal Methods

Non-hormonal methods are gaining attention due to the potential for fewer systemic side effects.

These include agents that interfere with sperm motility, maturation, or the ability to fertilize an egg without altering hormone levels. A prominent example is the drug candidate called Adjudin, which disrupts the adhesion of developing sperm cells to the Sertoli cells in the testes, effectively halting sperm production. Another is the reversible inhibition of sperm under guidance (RISUG), a polymer gel injected into the vas deferens that immobilizes sperm; it is undergoing advanced trials in India. The U.S. counterpart to this is Vasalgel, a similar hydrogel being studied as a long-acting, reversible male contraceptive.

Other Methods

Additional categories include retinoic acid receptor antagonists, which block vitamin A pathways essential for sperm production, and ion channel blockers like CatSper inhibitors that interfere with calcium signaling crucial to sperm motility. These drugs are still largely in experimental phases.

Unlike the wide array of female options, male contraceptive drugs are still emerging and mostly in trial stages. Condoms and vasectomy remain the only approved and widely used male-directed contraceptive methods, but drug-based alternatives may soon offer reversible, reliable options for men seeking to share in family planning responsibility.

Regarding male contraception, certain Ayurvedic antifertility herbs such as Guduchi (Tinospora cordifolia), Neem (Azadirachta indica), and Pippali (Piper longum) have demonstrated spermatotoxic or anti-implantation effects in animal models, suggesting that they might enhance contraceptive efficacy or serve as stand-alone agents in herbal male contraception if standardized properly.

Their interaction with pharmaceutical agents, however, remains under-studied and warrants caution. Conversely, rasayanas like Ashwagandha (Withania somnifera) and Kapikacchu (Mucuna pruriens) are known to enhance testosterone and sperm production, potentially counteracting the effects of testosterone-based contraceptives under investigation.

CANCER TREATMENT DRUGS

Cancer treatment has evolved significantly over the past several decades, expanding beyond traditional chemotherapy to include a wide range of pharmacological approaches. Each class of anti-cancer drugs works through distinct mechanisms and is often tailored to the type of cancer, the molecular profile of the tumor, and patient-specific factors. The major classes include chemotherapeutic agents, targeted therapies, hormonal therapies, immunotherapies, and several other emerging groups of drugs. Below is a comprehensive exploration of each of these classes.

Chemotherapy

Chemotherapy remains one of the most widely used treatments for cancer and includes drugs that broadly target rapidly dividing cells. These agents are cytotoxic, meaning they kill cells, particularly those that divide more frequently than normal—such as cancer cells. However, their lack of specificity also affects normal rapidly dividing cells (like those in the bone marrow, hair follicles, and gastrointestinal tract), leading to well-known side effects such as immunosuppression, alopecia, and nausea.

Chemotherapeutic drugs are categorized by their chemical structure and mechanism of action. Alkylating agents (e.g., cyclophosphamide, ifosfamide, and cisplatin) work by cross-linking DNA strands, thereby preventing replication. Antimetabolites (such as methotrexate, 5-fluorouracil, and gemcitabine) mimic natural substances within the cell, interfering with DNA and RNA synthesis. Mitotic inhibitors like paclitaxel and vincristine disrupt microtubule function, arresting cells during mitosis. Topoisomerase inhibitors, including doxorubicin and etoposide, prevent the uncoiling and re-coiling of DNA during replication. These drugs are often used in combination regimens to maximize cancer cell kill and minimize resistance.

Targeted Therapies

Targeted therapies are a more recent class of anti-cancer drugs that interfere with specific molecular targets involved in cancer growth and progression. These drugs are designed based on the understanding of genetic mutations or aberrant protein expressions that drive cancer. Unlike chemotherapy, which affects both cancerous and healthy cells, targeted therapy aims to specifically disrupt cancer cell pathways, leading to potentially fewer side effects.

There are several subclasses of targeted therapies. Tyrosine kinase inhibitors (TKIs) such as imatinib, erlotinib, and osimertinib block enzymes responsible for signal transduction involved in cell proliferation. Monoclonal antibodies like trastuzumab (targeting HER2 in breast cancer) or cetuximab (targeting EGFR in colorectal cancer) bind to specific antigens on cancer cells or in the tumor microenvironment. Other targeted agents include PARP inhibitors (e.g., olaparib for BRCA-mutated cancers) and angiogenesis inhibitors like bevacizumab, which inhibit the formation of new blood vessels needed to sustain tumor growth. These drugs are often used based on molecular diagnostics, such as next-generation sequencing, which guides personalized cancer therapy.

Hormone Therapies

Hormonal therapies are used in cancers that are hormone-sensitive, particularly breast, prostate, ovarian, and endometrial cancers. These cancers depend on hormones such as estrogen, progesterone, or androgens to grow. Hormonal therapy aims to block the body's ability to produce these hormones or to interfere with their effect on cancer cells.

In breast cancer, drugs like tamoxifen (a selective estrogen receptor modulator or SERM) and aromatase inhibitors (letrozole, anastrozole) either block estrogen receptors or reduce estrogen production. In prostate cancer, androgen deprivation therapy (ADT) is a cornerstone of treatment. This includes GnRH agonists (leuprolide, goserelin) that suppress testosterone production, and anti-androgens (enzalutamide, bicalutamide) that block androgen receptors. These treatments can be used alone or in combination with other therapies depending on disease stage and aggressiveness.

Immunotherapy

Immunotherapy represents a paradigm shift in cancer treatment, harnessing the body's immune system to recognize and attack cancer cells. These therapies aim to overcome the immune evasion tactics employed by tumors. Checkpoint inhibitors are the most widely used immunotherapies and work by releasing the "brakes" on immune cells. Drugs like pembrolizumab and nivolumab (anti-PD-1), atezolizumab (anti-PD-L1), and ipilimumab (anti-CTLA-4) enhance T-cell activity against tumors.

Other forms of immunotherapy include cancer vaccines, adoptive cell transfer (such as CAR T-cell therapy), and cytokine therapies (e.g., interleukin-2, interferons). CAR T-cell therapy, for example, involves engineering a patient's own T-cells to express receptors that recognize specific cancer antigens (such as CD19 in B-cell leukemia). While highly effective in some hematologic cancers, immunotherapy may be less predictable in solid tumors and can cause immune-related adverse events, such as colitis, pneumonitis, or endocrinopathies due to immune system overactivation.

Other Classes and Novel Approaches

Beyond the main categories, several other classes of anti-cancer drugs are emerging. Radiopharmaceuticals, such as radium-223 for prostate cancer with bone metastases, deliver radioactive isotopes directly to tumor sites. Epigenetic modulators, like histone deacetylase inhibitors (vorinostat) or DNA methyltransferase inhibitors (azacitidine), work by altering gene expression in cancer cells. Proteasome inhibitors, such as bortezomib, are primarily used in multiple myeloma and inhibit protein degradation pathways, leading to cancer cell death.

Antibody-drug conjugates (ADCs) represent a hybrid between targeted therapy and chemotherapy. They consist of a monoclonal antibody linked to a potent cytotoxic drug. The antibody binds to a specific tumor antigen, is internalized by the cancer cell, and releases the cytotoxic agent intracellularly—examples include trastuzumab emtansine (T-DM1) and sacituzumab and govitecan.

Oncolytic virus therapy is another promising frontier, involving genetically engineered viruses that preferentially infect and kill cancer cells while stimulating an anti-tumor immune response. Talimogene laherparepvec (T-VEC), an oncolytic herpesvirus, is approved for advanced melanoma.

Cancer Drug – Herb Interactions

One of the primary concerns with herb-drug interactions in cancer therapy is the effect of certain herbs on liver enzymes, particularly those in the cytochrome P450 family. These enzymes are responsible for metabolizing many chemotherapy and targeted therapy drugs.

St. John's Wort, for instance, is a well-known inducer of CYP3A4, an enzyme that metabolizes a large number of anti-cancer drugs including irinotecan, imatinib, and docetaxel. Taking St. John's wort concurrently can lead to faster drug breakdown and reduced plasma levels, potentially rendering the cancer treatment less effective. Conversely, herbs/foods like Grapefruit or Goldenseal may inhibit these enzymes, leading to elevated drug levels and increased toxicity.

Another class of interactions involves the modulation of drug transport proteins such as P-glycoprotein, which affects how drugs are absorbed, distributed, and excreted. Herbs like Green Tea, Ginseng, and Turmeric have been shown in some studies to inhibit or induce P-glycoprotein activity, possibly altering the intracellular concentration of certain chemotherapy agents. For example, Green tea's catechins may interfere with bortezomib, a proteasome inhibitor used in multiple myeloma, by binding to the drug and reducing its cytotoxicity. This suggests that even seemingly benign herbal teas may not be safe in all contexts when combined with anti-cancer drugs.

Immunomodulatory herbs pose another challenge. Herbs such as Echinacea and Astragalus are commonly used to stimulate the immune system, but their effects in the context of immunotherapy drugs such as checkpoint inhibitors (like nivolumab or pembrolizumab) are not fully understood. There is concern that they could either enhance immune-related side effects or, paradoxically, dampen the intended therapeutic response. Additionally, some herbs with antioxidant properties, such as high-dose vitamin E or Curcumin, may interfere with chemotherapy or radiation therapy, which rely on oxidative stress to kill cancer cells. While the clinical relevance of this remains debated, caution is generally advised when using potent antioxidant supplements during active cancer treatment.

Bleeding risk is another area of concern, especially for patients on anti-coagulants or those receiving drugs that impair platelet function. Garlic, Ginkgo Biloba, and Ginseng are all known to affect blood clotting pathways and may increase the risk of hemorrhage when used with certain chemotherapy agents, targeted therapies like bevacizumab, or supportive medications such as low-molecular-weight heparins. Similarly, herbs with estrogenic activity, such as Black cohosh or Red Clover, may be problematic in hormone-sensitive cancers like breast or prostate cancer, potentially opposing the effects of hormonal therapies like tamoxifen or aromatase inhibitors.

Despite the potential for harm, not all herb-drug interactions are negative. Some herbs may help mitigate side effects of cancer treatment, such as ginger for chemotherapy-induced nausea or licorice (in its deglycyrrhizinated form) for oral mucositis. However, the difference between therapeutic benefit and dangerous interaction often lies in the dose, the form of the herb, the timing of administration, and the individual patient's metabolism. Because herbal preparations are not regulated with the same rigor as pharmaceuticals, variability in composition and potency can further complicate safety assessments.

The co-use of herbal supplements and anti-cancer drugs requires careful consideration and open dialogue between patients and healthcare providers. Patients may not always disclose their use of herbal products, assuming they are natural and therefore safe, but clinicians must proactively inquire and be equipped to assess potential risks. Ongoing research is essential to clarify which combinations are safe and which are not. Until clearer guidelines are established, caution, transparency, and personalized assessment remain the cornerstones of integrating herbal medicine with cancer pharmacotherapy.

Herbs of special concern in this regard include:

Amalaki (Emblica officinalis):
High antioxidant content may theoretically blunt the efficacy of oxidative stress-dependent treatments like radiation and certain chemotherapeutics.

Ashwagandha (Withania somnifera):
May stimulate the immune system, which can interfere with immunotherapy or provoke autoimmune side effects. It may also affect thyroid function and hepatic enzymes.

Black Cohosh (Cimicifuga racemosa):
is also best avoided for people with breast or uterine cancers for similar reasons.

Brahmi (Bacopa monnieri):
May alter neurotransmitter function and potentially interact with chemotherapy-induced neurotoxicity or drugs affecting the central nervous system.

Echinacea (Echinacea spp.):
Can overstimulate the immune system, which can be problematic during certain immunotherapies.

Garlic (Allium sativum):
In large amounts can increase bleeding risk, which is a concern for patients with low platelet counts or those undergoing surgery. Kava and valerian may interact with sedative medications and put additional stress on the liver.

Ginger (Zingiber officinalis):
In large amounts can increase bleeding risk, which is a concern for patients with low platelet counts or those undergoing surgery. Kava and valerian may interact with sedative medications and put additional stress on the liver.

Ginseng (Panax spp.):
May interfere with blood sugar levels and hormone-sensitive cancers due to its phytoestrogenic effects.

Green tea extract (Camellia sinensis):
Can impact how some chemotherapy agents work and may dysregulate liver function.

Guduchi (Tinospora coridfolia):
Acts as an immune enhancer, which could worsen autoimmune-like reactions triggered by immunotherapy or reduce therapeutic response in specific protocols.

Guggulu (Commiphora mukul):
A known inducer of CYP3A4, which may reduce the efficacy of certain chemotherapy drugs. It may also act as a mild blood thinner.

Kappiakchhu (Mucuna pruriens):
Contains L-DOPA, which can interfere with dopamine pathways, and may interact unpredictably with drugs that affect the nervous system or hormonal balance.

Licorice (Glycyrrhiza glabra):
Can raise blood pressure and potassium levels, interfere with corticosteroid metabolism, and has estrogenic effects that may affect hormone-sensitive tumors.

Milk Thistle (Silybum marianum):
Can alter how the liver processes chemotherapy drugs, which can reduce their effectiveness or increase toxicity. Feverfew can also increase bleeding risk and affect platelet function.

Neem (Azidirachta indica):
Has immunostimulant properties and potential liver enzyme modulation. It may interfere with immune checkpoint inhibitors or cause hepatotoxicity in rare cases.

Red Clover (Trifolium pratensa):
Should generally be avoided during cancer treatment, especially for people with hormone-sensitive cancers like breast, ovarian, or prostate cancer, because it contains phytoestrogens that can mimic estrogen in the body and potentially promote tumor growth or interfere with hormone therapies. Although it's sometimes marketed for

menopausal symptoms, its estrogen-like effects can be risky when cancer is involved.

St. John's Wort (Hypericum perforatum):
Should be avoided because it can interfere with the effectiveness of chemotherapy drugs by dysregulsting liver enzymes that metabolize medications.

Shatavari (Asparagus racemosus):
Contains phytoestrogens, making it potentially dangerous in hormone-sensitive cancers such as breast or prostate cancer.

Triphala: (Multiherbal ofmrula):
Can have mild laxative effects and may impair drug absorption. Amla (Emblica officinalis) itself has high antioxidant activity that could interfere with radiation or chemotherapy.

Tulsi (Ocimum sanctum):
Known for strong immunomodulatory and antioxidant properties, which may reduce the efficacy of therapies that induce reactive oxygen species (ROS).

Turmeric (Curcuma longa):
In higher doses can thin the blood and interact with chemotherapy drugs, although culinary amounts are usually fine. It also may act as an antioxidant and potentially reduce the oxidative damage that chemotherapy or radiation depends upon. It also interacts with several liver enzymes and drug transporters.

PRESCRIPTION VITAMINS AND MINERALS

Prescription vitamins and minerals are supplements that a healthcare provider may prescribe to treat or prevent deficiencies. These differ from over the counter (OTC) vitamins in that they often contain higher doses, are formulated for specific medical conditions, or are in a form that is more readily absorbed by the body. These prescription vitamins and minerals are usually tailored to the individual's needs based on their medical condition, lab results, and overall health status. The most commonly prescribed follow.

Vitamin D
Ergocalciferol (Vitamin D2): Used to treat Vitamin D deficiencies, often in patients with conditions like osteoporosis or chronic kidney disease. A commonly prescribed brand is *Drisdol*.
Cholecalciferol (Vitamin D3): Another form of Vitamin D prescribed for deficiencies, particularly when high doses are required.
A commonly prescribed brand is *Calciferol*.

Vitamin B12
Cyanocobalamin: Often prescribed for people with B12 deficiency due to conditions like pernicious anemia, or absorption issues related to gastric surgery. A frequently prescribed brand is *Nascobal*.
Methylcobalamin: A form of B12 that is sometimes preferred due to its higher bioavailability.
A frequently prescribed brand is *Mecobalamin*.

Folic Acid (Vitamin B9)

Folic Acid Tablets: Prescribed to prevent neural tube defects in pregnancy, and to treat folic acid deficiency anemia.
Frequently prescribed brands are *Folacin -800* and *Folvite*.

Vitamin A
Retinoic Acid: Sometimes prescribed in high doses for conditions like acne or other skin disorders. Commonly prescribed forms include *Renova, Avita,* and *Atralin*
A water-miscible form of Vitamin A, often prescribed for patients with fat malabsorption disorders is sold as *Aquasol A:*.

Iron Supplements
Ferrous Sulfate: Commonly prescribed for iron deficiency anemia. Commonly prescribed forms are *Slow FE* and *Ferotab*.
Ferrous Gluconate: Another form of iron that may be prescribed, especially if the patient experiences gastrointestinal issues with ferrous sulfate.
Commonly prescribed forms are *Ferate* and *Fergon*.

Calcium
Calcium Carbonate: Prescribed for calcium deficiency, often in patients with osteoporosis or those at risk for osteoporosis. A commonly prescribed form is *Calcitriol*.
Calcium Citrate: Preferred for patients who need to avoid excess stomach acid. A frequently used brand is *Caltrate.*

Magnesium
Magnesium Oxide: Prescribed to treat magnesium deficiency, which can occur in patients taking certain diuretics or with chronic gastrointestinal disorders.

Frequently used brands are *MagOx* and *Magoxide.*
Magnesium Sulfate: Sometimes used in intravenous form for severe deficiencies or specific conditions like preeclampsia. MgSO4 or Epsom Salt is widely available under a wide variety of names.

Zinc
Zinc Sulfate: Prescribed to treat zinc deficiency, which can impair immune function and wound healing. Frequently used brand are *ZN-500* and *Zincate*

Potassium
Potassium Chloride: Often prescribed for patients with hypokalemia (low potassium levels), which can occur due to diuretics or certain medical conditions. A widely used prescription brand is *Evion.*

Prenatal Vitamins
Prescription Prenatal Vitamins: These often contain higher doses of folic acid, iron, and other essential nutrients compared to non-prescription versions, and are tailored for pregnant women. Common prescription brands are *Pre-Nexa* and *PrenaPlus.*

Vitamin E
Alpha-tocopherol: Prescribed in certain conditions where there is a documented deficiency, or for specific neurological disorders. A widely used prescription brand is *Evion.*

Vitamin K
Phytonadione (Vitamin K1): Used to treat or prevent bleeding disorders associated with Vitamin K deficiency,

particularly in newborns or patients on anticoagulant therapy. A widely used prescription brand is *Mephyton*.

Chapter 4:
HERB-DRUG INTERACTIONS

The following are the most widely prescribed pharmaceutical drugs in the US nd Canada, along with their most widely sold brand names, and listing with each herbal substances with the capacity of interacting.

Herb-drug interactions can be complex, and the effects may vary depending on individual health conditions and other medications being taken. This list may change as new drugs enter the market and prescription trends evolve.

For many of these drugs there are no interactions that are known; the fact that there are no known herbal interactions does not in any way convey that they do not have such interactions. Research in this area is continuing, and without doubt there are interactions yet to be uncovered.

This list includes a variety of medications for different conditions, including cardiovascular diseases, mental health disorders, infections, and chronic diseases.

The following list is arranged alphabetically.

Acetaminophen (*Tylenol, Paracetamol*), a widely used analgesic and antipyretic, is generally considered safe when taken at recommended doses, but it can interact with a variety of Western and Ayurvedic herbs that affect liver metabolism, antioxidant capacity, or detoxification pathways.

Because Acetaminophen is metabolized primarily in the liver through conjugation and cytochrome P450 enzymes (especially CYP2E1), concurrent use of herbs that induce or inhibit these enzymes—such as St. John's Wort, Goldenseal, Grapefruit, and in Ayurveda, Pippali, Tulsi, and Licorice—may alter the rate of metabolism, potentially increasing the risk of liver toxicity or reducing the drug's effectiveness.

High doses or prolonged use of Acetaminophen can deplete glutathione and cause oxidative stress in the liver, so antioxidant and hepatoprotective herbs like Milk Thistle, Bhumyamalaki, Amalaki, and Guduchi may offer protective benefits when used cautiously and spaced from dosing.

Herbs with mild analgesic or anti-inflammatory effects—such as Turmeric, Ginger, Boswellia (Shallaki), and Willow Bark—may enhance pain relief but should be used carefully to avoid unintentional overmedication or added strain on the liver.

Laxative or diuretic herbs such as Senna, Aloe, Punarnava, and Dandelion may influence hydration and detoxification processes, potentially affecting how the body handles Acetaminophen's metabolites.

Although Acetaminophen does not have significant blood-thinning or sedative properties, it is often combined with other medications that do, and this can amplify risks when taken with herbs that affect clotting, such as Garlic or Guggulu, or herbs that calm the nervous system, such as Valerian or Ashwagandha.

Because liver damage is the most serious risk associated with Acetaminophen—especially when combined with alcohol or other hepatotoxic substances—any regular use of herbal supplements should be reviewed with a healthcare provider to ensure safe dosing and avoid interactions that could compromise liver function.

Albuterol (*Ventolin, ProAir, Proventil*) a fast-acting beta-2 adrenergic agonist used primarily for the relief of bronchospasm in asthma, chronic obstructive pulmonary disease (COPD), and exercise-induced bronchoconstriction, can interact with various Western and Ayurvedic herbs that affect the respiratory system, cardiovascular function, nervous system stimulation, or electrolyte balance.

Because Albuterol stimulates beta receptors to relax airway muscles and improve breathing, combining it with stimulant herbs—such as Ephedra, Guarana, Yohimbe, and in Ayurveda, Vacha, Bala, and Shilajit—can intensify its effects on heart rate, blood pressure, and nervous system activity, potentially leading to palpitations, tremors, anxiety, or insomnia.

Conversely, calming and antispasmodic herbs like Lobelia, Mullein, Skullcap, Passionflower, and in Ayurveda, Jatamansi, Ashwagandha, and Shankhapushpi may counterbalance overstimulation and support relaxation of respiratory pathways.

Albuterol can cause mild to moderate shifts in potassium levels, so the use of laxative or diuretic herbs such as Senna, Aloe, Dandelion, Uva Ursi, or Punarnava may exacerbate hypokalemia, increasing the risk of muscle cramps, weakness, or arrhythmias, especially in high or prolonged doses.

Although Albuterol is not heavily metabolized by the liver, herbs that influence adrenal or cardiovascular function—such as Licorice, Ginseng, Hawthorn, or Arjuna—may still impact its physiologic effects, either enhancing or opposing its bronchodilatory and stimulant actions. Immune-supportive herbs like Echinacea, Astragalus, Amalaki, and Tulsi are often used during respiratory infections and may be helpful adjuncts if timed appropriately and monitored for any overstimulation or herb-drug synergy.

Because Albuterol has rapid onset and dose-sensitive cardiovascular side effects, the use of herbal supplements—especially those with stimulant or fluid-altering properties—should be approached with caution and discussed with a healthcare provider, particularly in individuals with cardiovascular sensitivity or electrolyte imbalances.

Allopurinol (Zyloprim, Aloprim), a xanthine oxidase inhibitor used to lower uric acid levels in conditions such as gout, kidney stones, and tumor lysis syndrome, can interact with several Western and Ayurvedic herbs that affect purine metabolism, liver detoxification, renal function, or inflammation.

Because Allopurinol reduces uric acid production, combining it with uric acid–modifying or diuretic herbs—such as Nettle, Celery Seed, Dandelion, Uva Ursi, and in Ayurveda, Punarnava, Gokshura, and Varuna—may enhance its uricosuric effects, potentially improving outcomes but also increasing the risk of electrolyte imbalance or kidney irritation if not properly dosed. Anti-inflammatory herbs commonly used for gout—such as Turmeric, Ginger, Boswellia (Shallaki), and Willow Bark—may complement Allopurinol's role in managing flare-ups, but excessive or unmonitored use could increase gastrointestinal burden or interact with other medications used during acute attacks.

Allopurinol is metabolized in the liver and excreted through the kidneys, so herbs that affect liver enzymes such as St. John's Wort, Goldenseal, Grapefruit, and in Ayurveda, Pippali, Tulsi, and Bhumyamalaki may alter its metabolism or the metabolism of other drugs taken with it.

Herbal laxatives like Senna or Aloe may contribute to dehydration and strain kidney function, which can affect Allopurinol excretion and increase the risk of toxicity.

Immunomodulating herbs like Echinacea, Astragalus, Ashwagandha, and Amalaki may either support immune function or, in rare cases, interfere with hypersensitivity reactions associated with Allopurinol, which can be serious.

Because Allopurinol carries a risk of rare but potentially severe side effects such as Stevens-Johnson syndrome or liver toxicity, the use of herbal supplements—especially those affecting detoxification pathways, hydration, or immune response—should be done cautiously and under the guidance of a qualified practitioner.

Alprazolam (*Xanax, Xanax XR*), a short-acting benzodiazepine used to treat anxiety, panic disorder, and occasionally insomnia, has a high potential for interactions with Western and Ayurvedic herbs that affect sedation, liver metabolism, or mood regulation.

Because Alprazolam acts on GABA-A receptors to produce calming and anxiolytic effects, combining it with sedative or nervine herbs—such as Valerian, Kava, Skullcap, Lemon Balm, Chamomile, Passionflower, and Hops—can significantly increase central nervous system depression, leading to excessive drowsiness, confusion, poor coordination, or even respiratory suppression in vulnerable individuals.

Similarly, Ayurvedic herbs like Ashwagandha, Jatamansi, Tagara, Shankhapushpi, and Brahmi may have synergistic calming effects that intensify Alprazolam's action, especially when used in high doses or combined formulations.

Alprazolam is primarily metabolized by the liver enzyme CYP3A4, making it susceptible to interactions with herbs such as St. John's Wort, which may reduce its effectiveness by inducing metabolism, and Grapefruit, Goldenseal, and Ayurvedic agents like Tulsi, Pippali, and Licorice, which may inhibit metabolism and raise drug levels, increasing the risk of adverse effects.

Stimulating herbs such as Ephedra, Guarana, Yohimbe, and Vacha may antagonize the calming effects of Alprazolam, potentially leading to increased anxiety, agitation, or restlessness.

Laxative or diuretic herbs like Senna, Aloe, Dandelion, and Punarnava may influence fluid and electrolyte balance, which could worsen symptoms like lightheadedness or fatigue, especially in those sensitive to changes in blood pressure or hydration.

Because Alprazolam has a short half-life, risk of dependence, and a strong impact on mental clarity and alertness, the use of any herbal supplements should be carefully reviewed and ideally supervised by a healthcare provider familiar with the potential for additive sedation, altered metabolism, or withdrawal complications.

Amlodipine (*Norvasc, Katerzia, Norliqva*) a long-acting calcium channel blocker used to treat high blood pressure and angina, may interact with a variety of Western and Ayurvedic herbs that affect vascular tone, sedation, liver metabolism, or fluid balance.

Herbs with blood pressure–lowering effects—such as Hawthorn, Garlic, Motherwort, and in Ayurveda, Arjuna, Sarpagandha, Ashwagandha, and Jatamansi—can enhance the hypotensive action of Amlodipine, potentially leading to dizziness, fainting, or lightheadedness, particularly when changing position or in combination with diuretics.

Sedative and calming herbs like Valerian, Skullcap, Kava, Lemon Balm, Passionflower, and in Ayurveda, Tagara, Shankhapushpi, and Brahmi, may further contribute to fatigue or low energy when used with Amlodipine, especially in sensitive individuals.

Amlodipine is metabolized primarily through the liver enzyme CYP3A4, making it vulnerable to interactions with herbs that affect this pathway. St. John's Wort may reduce Amlodipine's effectiveness by speeding up its metabolism, while Grapefruit, Goldenseal, and Ayurvedic agents like Pippali, Tulsi, and Licorice may inhibit metabolism and increase drug levels, heightening the risk of side effects such as peripheral edema, flushing, or palpitations.

Diuretic or detoxifying herbs like Dandelion, Punarnava, and Gokshura may alter fluid and electrolyte balance and could intensify blood pressure changes or swelling in certain individuals.

Although Amlodipine does not typically cause electrolyte disturbances, herbs that affect potassium or sodium levels may still influence cardiovascular stability when used concurrently. Because Amlodipine is often used long-term and has a slow onset and extended duration of action, herbal combinations should be approached thoughtfully, with attention to blood pressure trends, fatigue, and fluid retention, and preferably with the guidance of a qualified healthcare provider.

Amoxicillin (*Amoxil, Trimox*), a widely used penicillin-class antibiotic, is generally well tolerated and has a low risk of serious herb-drug interactions, but certain Western and Ayurvedic herbs may still affect its absorption, efficacy, or the body's response to treatment.

Because Amoxicillin is absorbed through the gastrointestinal tract, herbs with high tannin or mineral content—such as Alfalfa, Horsetail, Nettle, Triphala, and Guduchi—may bind to the drug and reduce its effectiveness if taken at the same time.

Laxative or purgative herbs like Senna, Aloe, Cascara, and Punarnava may exacerbate gastrointestinal side effects such as diarrhea, cramping, or nausea, which are already common with Amoxicillin.

On the other hand, demulcent and gut-soothing herbs like Slippery Elm, Marshmallow Root, Licorice, Yashtimadhu, and Shatavari may help protect the digestive lining and reduce discomfort, especially if taken separately from the antibiotic.

Although Amoxicillin is not significantly metabolized by liver enzymes such as CYP450, herbs that support or burden detoxification pathways—like Milk Thistle, Dandelion Root, Bhumyamalaki, and Tulsi—may still influence the body's overall ability to handle the drug and its metabolites.

Immune-supporting herbs such as Echinacea, Astragalus, Ashwagandha, and Amalaki may complement the antibiotic's effect when used appropriately, although overstimulation of the immune system during infection may cause unpredictable reactions.

Antimicrobial herbs such as Goldenseal, Oregon Grape, Neem, Garlic, and Turmeric may either assist or interfere with Amoxicillin's action depending on dosage, timing, and the state of the microbiome.

As with all antibiotics, preservation of gut flora is important, and probiotic-rich foods or herbal support may help restore balance during and after treatment.
While Amoxicillin is one of the more herb-compatible antibiotics, herbal supplements should still be spaced apart from doses and selected with care, especially in individuals with sensitive digestion or chronic health conditions.

Apixaban (*Eliquis*) an oral anticoagulant that directly inhibits factor Xa, is used to prevent and treat blood clots in conditions such as atrial fibrillation, deep vein thrombosis, and pulmonary embolism, and it carries a high risk of herb interactions, particularly with herbs that affect coagulation, liver metabolism, or renal clearance.
Because Apixaban reduces the blood's ability to clot, combining it with anticoagulant or antiplatelet herbs—such as Garlic, Ginger, Ginkgo, Turmeric, Willow Bark, and in Ayurveda, Guggulu, Haridra, Arjuna, and Shallaki—may significantly increase the risk of bruising, bleeding gums, nosebleeds, gastrointestinal bleeding, or more serious hemorrhagic events.
Although Apixaban is not a substrate of CYP enzymes to the same extent as some other drugs, it is metabolized in part by CYP3A4 and is a known substrate of P-glycoprotein, meaning that herbs such as St. John's Wort (which induces both pathways) may reduce its effectiveness, while inhibitors like Grapefruit, Goldenseal, and in Ayurveda, Pippali, Tulsi, and Licorice may increase blood levels and bleeding risk.
Diuretic or detoxifying herbs like Dandelion, Uva Ursi, Punarnava, and Gokshura can affect renal function and fluid balance, which may indirectly influence drug

clearance, especially in older adults or those with compromised kidney function.

Some soothing or anti-inflammatory herbs such as Chamomile, Boswellia, or Ashwagandha may be compatible but still carry mild anticoagulant or immunomodulatory properties that could compound Apixaban's effects in sensitive individuals.

Because Apixaban has no easily reversible antidote outside of specialized settings and because even minor herbal additions can tip the balance toward dangerous bleeding, any use of herbal supplements—especially those affecting circulation, inflammation, or liver enzymes—should be undertaken with great caution and only under supervision.

Aripiprazole (*Abilify, Aristada*), an atypical antipsychotic used to treat conditions such as schizophrenia, bipolar disorder, major depressive disorder, and irritability associated with autism, has a complex pharmacologic profile and may interact with a variety of Western and Ayurvedic herbs that influence dopamine, serotonin, sedation, or liver enzyme activity.

Aripiprazole acts as a partial agonist at dopamine D2 and serotonin 5-HT1A receptors, and an antagonist at 5-HT2A receptors, which means that herbs with serotonergic or dopaminergic activity—such as St. John's Wort, Mucuna Pruriens, Rhodiola, and in Ayurveda, Kapikacchu, Ashwagandha, and Shankhapushpi—can influence mood or behavior in ways that may either complement or destabilize its effects.

Because Aripiprazole can cause sedation or agitation depending on the individual, combining it with calming herbs like Valerian, Skullcap, Lemon Balm, Chamomile, Jatamansi, Tagara, or Brahmi may increase drowsiness or

dull mental clarity, while stimulating herbs like Guarana, Ephedra, Yohimbe, and Vacha may heighten restlessness, anxiety, or insomnia.
Aripiprazole is primarily metabolized by CYP2D6 and CYP3A4 enzymes, making it vulnerable to interactions with herbs such as Grapefruit, Goldenseal, Milk Thistle, and Ayurvedic agents like Pippali, Tulsi, and Licorice, which may inhibit or alter its breakdown and affect blood levels of the drug.
Conversely, St. John's Wort may induce these enzymes and lower Aripiprazole concentrations, reducing its therapeutic effect.
Since Aripiprazole can affect impulse control and mood stability, herbs with psychoactive or mood-altering properties—even if mild—should be approached cautiously.
Herbal supplements that affect blood sugar or weight, such as Guggulu or Fenugreek, may also influence Aripiprazole's metabolic side effects.
Given its long half-life, dopamine-related effects, and individualized response profile, any herbal use alongside Aripiprazole should be carefully considered and monitored by a healthcare professional familiar with both psychiatric medications and herbal medicine.

Aspirin (*Bayer Aspirin, Ecotrin*), a nonsteroidal anti-inflammatory drug (NSAID) with antiplatelet properties, is widely used for pain relief, inflammation, fever reduction, and cardiovascular prevention, but it interacts with many Western and Ayurvedic herbs that influence blood clotting, gastrointestinal health, and renal function.
Because Aspirin irreversibly inhibits platelet aggregation, herbs with natural blood-thinning effects—such as Garlic, Ginger, Ginkgo, Turmeric, Willow Bark, Feverfew, and in

Ayurveda, Guggulu, Haridra, Arjuna, and Shallaki—can significantly increase the risk of bruising, bleeding gums, gastrointestinal bleeding, or even hemorrhagic stroke when taken concurrently.

Aspirin is also harsh on the gastric mucosa, so combining it with irritant or laxative herbs such as Senna, Aloe, Cascara, and Punarnava may further increase the risk of gastritis, ulcers, or bleeding.

Soothing, demulcent herbs like Slippery Elm, Licorice, Marshmallow Root, and Shatavari may be helpful in protecting the stomach lining and reducing discomfort when taken at a separate time from the medication.

Although Aspirin is not heavily dependent on liver metabolism, herbs that affect liver enzymes such as St. John's Wort, Goldenseal, and in Ayurveda, Pippali and Tulsi, may still interfere with the metabolism of other medications taken alongside Aspirin.

Kidney function is also a concern, especially in long-term users, and combining Aspirin with diuretic or nephrotoxic herbs like Dandelion, Uva Ursi, and Gokshura may further burden renal filtration.

Because Aspirin's antiplatelet effect lasts for the life of the platelet (around 7–10 days), even intermittent herb use during Aspirin therapy can have cumulative effects on bleeding risk.

For patients using Aspirin regularly, especially in cardiovascular or post-stroke care, herbal supplements should be chosen with great care and preferably under the guidance of a knowledgeable healthcare provider.

Atorvastatin (*Lipitor, Atorvaliq*), a statin medication used to lower cholesterol and reduce cardiovascular risk, can interact with a range of Western and Ayurvedic herbs that affect liver metabolism, lipid levels, antioxidant pathways, or muscle health.

Atorvastatin is metabolized primarily by the liver enzyme CYP3A4, making it susceptible to interference from herbs such as St. John's Wort, which may reduce its effectiveness by inducing the enzyme, and Grapefruit, Goldenseal, and in Ayurveda, Pippali, Tulsi, and Licorice, which may inhibit metabolism and increase blood levels, raising the risk of side effects like muscle pain or liver enzyme elevation.

Some herbs used to lower cholesterol—such as Red Yeast Rice, Garlic, Gugulipid (Guggulu), Fenugreek, and Turmeric—may have additive lipid-lowering effects, which can be beneficial but may also increase the risk of liver strain or gastrointestinal discomfort when used together with Atorvastatin.

Antioxidant-rich herbs such as Milk Thistle, Green Tea, Amalaki, and Haridra may support liver and cardiovascular health, but high doses could theoretically reduce the drug's mild pro-oxidant effect that contributes to its plaque-stabilizing action.

Myopathy and muscle-related side effects are a known risk of statins, and this risk may be heightened by combining Atorvastatin with herbs that deplete coenzyme Q10 or interfere with mitochondrial function, such as high-dose Red Yeast Rice or Policosanol.

Ayurvedic herbs like Ashwagandha, Shatavari, and Triphala are often used to support overall cardiovascular and liver function and are generally safe when used appropriately and spaced apart from dosing.

Because Atorvastatin is used long-term and affects multiple systems—including liver, muscle, and metabolism—herbal combinations should be evaluated carefully and adjusted in consultation with a healthcare provider to ensure safety and effectiveness.

Azithromycin (*Zithromax, Zmax*), a macrolide antibiotic used to treat respiratory, skin, and sexually transmitted infections, generally has a moderate interaction profile but can still be affected by various Western and Ayurvedic herbs that influence gastrointestinal function, liver enzymes, or microbial balance.
Although Azithromycin is not heavily dependent on cytochrome P450 enzymes like some other macrolides, it is a mild inhibitor of CYP3A4 and P-glycoprotein, so herbs such as St. John's Wort, Goldenseal, Grapefruit, and in Ayurveda, Pippali, Tulsi, and Licorice may alter its activity or the levels of other medications taken concurrently.
Herbs with antimicrobial effects—such as Garlic, Oregano Oil, Echinacea, Goldenseal, Neem, and Turmeric—may have overlapping or antagonistic effects, and when used in excess, could disrupt microbial balance or increase the risk of resistance.
In Ayurveda, Amalaki, Haridra, and Triphala may offer supportive immune or detoxifying effects but should be spaced a few hours from antibiotic dosing to avoid interference with absorption.
Azithromycin is known for gastrointestinal side effects such as nausea, diarrhea, or cramping, which may be worsened by laxative or irritant herbs like Senna, Aloe, Cascara, and Punarnava.
Conversely, soothing demulcent herbs like Slippery Elm, Marshmallow Root, and Licorice, or Ayurvedic agents like Yashtimadhu and Shatavari, may help reduce gut irritation when used away from the drug.
Because Azithromycin has a long half-life and a broad spectrum of activity, preserving gut flora during and after

treatment is important, and overuse of antimicrobial or immune-stimulating herbs during therapy may disrupt recovery.

While Azithromycin is generally well-tolerated, herb-drug interactions—especially involving the gut, immune system, or metabolism—should still be managed thoughtfully, with attention to spacing, dosage, and the individual's digestive sensitivity.

Baclofen (*Lioresal, Gablofen*), a centrally acting skeletal muscle relaxant used to treat spasticity in conditions such as multiple sclerosis and spinal cord injury, works primarily by enhancing GABA-B receptor activity in the spinal cord and brain, and it can interact with a number of Western and Ayurvedic herbs that affect the nervous system, muscle tone, or kidney function.

Herbs with sedative, antispasmodic, or nervine properties—including Valerian, Kava, Skullcap, Lemon Balm, Passionflower, and Chamomile—may amplify Baclofen's central nervous system depressant effects, increasing the risk of excessive drowsiness, dizziness, slowed reflexes, and in rare cases, respiratory depression. Ayurvedic herbs such as Ashwagandha, Tagara, Jatamansi, Shankhapushpi, and Brahmi may exert similar calming and muscle-relaxing effects and could act synergistically, potentially leading to oversedation or muscle weakness.

Baclofen is excreted primarily through the kidneys, so herbs with diuretic or renal-stimulating effects—such as Dandelion, Uva Ursi, Juniper, and in Ayurveda, Punarnava and Gokshura—may alter the elimination of the drug, potentially affecting its plasma levels or duration of action. Although Baclofen is not heavily dependent on liver metabolism, herbs that alter the nervous system balance,

such as stimulant herbs like Ephedra, Guarana, Yohimbe, and Vacha, may oppose its effects, increasing muscle tension, anxiety, or nervous system irritability.
Laxative herbs like Senna or Aloe could also influence electrolyte levels, which may further affect neuromuscular function when used in combination with Baclofen.
Because Baclofen can cause withdrawal symptoms if abruptly discontinued and may lead to sedation, hypotonia, or confusion at higher doses, herbal supplements should be introduced cautiously and always under professional supervision, particularly in patients with compromised renal function or concurrent CNS medications.

Bupropion (*Wellbutrin, Aplenzin, Zyban, Forfivo XL*), is an atypical antidepressant and smoking cessation aid that acts primarily by inhibiting the reuptake of norepinephrine and dopamine, and it can interact with a variety of Western and Ayurvedic herbs that influence neurotransmitters, liver enzymes, or seizure threshold. Unlike SSRIs and SNRIs, Bupropion does not significantly affect serotonin, but it lowers the seizure threshold, making interactions with stimulant or pro-convulsant herbs especially concerning.
Herbs with stimulating effects—such as Ephedra, Yohimbe, Guarana, Green Tea, and in Ayurveda, Vacha, Bala, and Shilajit—may increase the risk of anxiety, insomnia, restlessness, or even seizures when combined with Bupropion.
Sedative or calming herbs like Valerian, Skullcap, Passionflower, Kava, and in Ayurveda, Ashwagandha, Jatamansi, Tagara, and Shankhapushpi may either help offset these effects or contribute to unpredictable nervous system responses, depending on individual sensitivity.

Bupropion is metabolized primarily by the liver enzyme CYP2B6, so herbs that affect hepatic enzymes—such as St. John's Wort (a potent inducer) or Grapefruit, Goldenseal, and Ayurvedic herbs like Pippali, Tulsi, and Licorice (potential inhibitors)—may alter Bupropion's levels in the bloodstream, either reducing its effectiveness or increasing the risk of side effects.

Because Bupropion carries a black box warning for increased seizure risk at higher doses or when combined with other pro-convulsant substances, additional caution is warranted when using herbs with stimulant, laxative, or electrolyte-depleting properties such as Senna, Aloe, or Punarnava, which may further lower the seizure threshold. Unlike serotonergic drugs, Bupropion does not typically interact with serotonin-boosting herbs like 5-HTP or SAMe, but mood-enhancing adaptogens like Rhodiola, Ginseng, and Mucuna Pruriens should still be used carefully due to potential overlaps in dopaminergic effects. Given its distinct mechanism and seizure risk, combining Bupropion with herbs should be done only under the guidance of a knowledgeable healthcare provider.

Carvedilol (*Coreg, Coreg CR*), a non-selective beta-blocker with additional alpha-blocking activity, is commonly prescribed for hypertension, heart failure, and post–myocardial infarction management, and it can interact with various Western and Ayurvedic herbs that influence cardiovascular function, blood pressure, sedation, or liver metabolism.

Herbs with hypotensive effects—such as Hawthorn, Garlic, Motherwort, and in Ayurveda, Arjuna, Sarpagandha, Ashwagandha, and Jatamansi—can enhance the blood pressure–lowering effects of Carvedilol, increasing the risk of dizziness, lightheadedness, or fainting, especially when rising from a seated position.

Sedative herbs such as Valerian, Skullcap, Lemon Balm, Passionflower, and Kava may also amplify Carvedilol's fatigue-inducing and bradycardic effects, leading to excessive drowsiness or slowed heart rate. Ayurvedic herbs like Tagara, Shankhapushpi, and Brahmi may have similar synergistic effects on the nervous system.

Carvedilol is metabolized in the liver primarily through the CYP2D6 and CYP2C9 enzyme systems, which means that herbs like St. John's Wort can reduce its effectiveness by inducing these enzymes, while Goldenseal, Grapefruit, and Ayurvedic herbs like Pippali, Tulsi, and Licorice may inhibit metabolism, leading to increased plasma levels and side effects such as hypotension or bradycardia.

Stimulant herbs such as Ephedra, Yohimbe, Guarana, and Vacha may antagonize Carvedilol's action by raising blood pressure or heart rate, increasing cardiovascular stress and reducing the drug's efficacy.

Diuretic or detoxifying herbs like Dandelion, Punarnava, and Gokshura may affect fluid balance and kidney function, which can be relevant in heart failure patients taking Carvedilol.

Because this drug is often used in vulnerable cardiac populations and has dose-dependent effects on both blood pressure and heart rate, herbal supplementation should be undertaken with careful monitoring and the involvement of a qualified healthcare provider.

Celecoxib (*Celebrex, Elyxyb*), a selective COX-2 inhibitor used to treat pain and inflammation in conditions like osteoarthritis, rheumatoid arthritis, and acute injury, can interact with various Western and Ayurvedic herbs that influence blood clotting, gastrointestinal health, liver metabolism, or renal function.

Although Celecoxib has a lower risk of gastrointestinal bleeding compared to non-selective NSAIDs, combining it with herbs that thin the blood—such as Garlic, Ginkgo, Ginger, Turmeric, and Willow Bark—may increase the risk of bleeding, especially in older adults or those on other anticoagulants.

Similarly, Ayurvedic herbs like Guggulu, Shallaki, Haridra, and Arjuna have mild antiplatelet effects and may compound this risk when used concurrently. Celecoxib is metabolized primarily by the liver enzyme CYP2C9, making it susceptible to interference by herbs such as St. John's Wort, which may reduce its effectiveness by inducing metabolism, and Goldenseal, Grapefruit, or in Ayurveda, Tulsi, Pippali, and Licorice, which may inhibit metabolism and increase plasma levels.

Kidney function can also be affected by Celecoxib, especially when combined with dehydrating or diuretic herbs like Dandelion, Uva Ursi, Juniper, and Punarnava, potentially increasing the risk of nephrotoxicity.

Some herbs used for joint pain or inflammation, such as Devil's Claw, Cat's Claw, Boswellia (Shallaki), and Ashwagandha, may either enhance or complicate Celecoxib's anti-inflammatory action, and should be monitored for additive effects.

While the gastrointestinal risk is lower with Celecoxib, prolonged use with irritant or laxative herbs like Senna, Aloe, and Cascara may still provoke discomfort or damage to the mucosal lining.

Because Celecoxib is often used long-term and interacts with multiple systems, concurrent use of herbal products should be discussed with a qualified practitioner, especially when bleeding risk, liver enzymes, or kidney function are of concern.

Cephalexin (*Keflex, Bio-Cef, Panixine*), a first-generation cephalosporin antibiotic used to treat bacterial infections of the skin, respiratory tract, urinary tract, and more, generally has a lower potential for herb-drug interactions than many other medications, but there are still important considerations involving both Western and Ayurvedic herbs.
Mineral-rich or tannin-containing herbs—such as Alfalfa, Horsetail, Nettle, Triphala, and Guduchi—may interfere with Cephalexin absorption when taken at the same time, potentially reducing its effectiveness.
Herbs that alter gastrointestinal function, such as Senna, Aloe, Cascara, and Punarnava, may cause diarrhea or disrupt the gut microbiome, which can already be affected by antibiotics, leading to an increased risk of digestive side effects.
Immune-modulating herbs like Echinacea, Astragalus, Ashwagandha, and Amalaki may be supportive during antibiotic treatment, but they can also affect the intensity or duration of the immune response and should be timed carefully.
Probiotic-supportive herbs and foods, such as Slippery Elm, Marshmallow Root, and Licorice, may help soothe antibiotic-induced irritation of the gut lining and are generally compatible when spaced a few hours apart.
Cephalexin is not heavily metabolized by the liver, so major cytochrome P450 interactions with herbs like St. John's Wort, Goldenseal, or Grapefruit are unlikely, but supportive herbs like Milk Thistle or Bhumyamalaki may still be used to promote general liver and immune health.
As with any antibiotic, preserving gut flora is key, so

caution is advised when using herbs with strong antimicrobial activity, including Oregon Grape, Goldenseal, Neem, and Turmeric, which might further disturb microbial balance if overused.

While Cephalexin is relatively herb-friendly compared to many other drugs, herbal supplements should still be used with care, ideally spaced apart from doses and selected based on an individual's digestive and immune response.

Clonazepam (*Klonopin, Rivotril*), a long-acting benzodiazepine used to treat anxiety, panic disorders, and certain types of seizures, has a high potential for interaction with Western and Ayurvedic herbs, especially those that affect the central nervous system, sedation, or liver metabolism.

Sedative and calming herbs—including Valerian, Kava, Hops, Skullcap, Chamomile, Passionflower, and Lemon Balm—can significantly enhance the depressant effects of Clonazepam, increasing the risk of excessive drowsiness, confusion, dizziness, impaired coordination, and respiratory depression.

Ayurvedic herbs such as Ashwagandha, Jatamansi, Tagara, Shankhapushpi, and Brahmi may also have synergistic effects on GABAergic pathways, intensifying the drug's action and side effects.

Clonazepam is primarily metabolized through the cytochrome P450 system, particularly CYP3A enzymes, making it susceptible to interactions with herbs that affect this pathway. St. John's Wort can reduce Clonazepam levels by inducing CYP3A4, potentially reducing its effectiveness, while herbs such as Grapefruit, Goldenseal, Milk Thistle, and Ayurvedic agents like Tulsi, Pippali, and Bhumyamalaki may inhibit these enzymes, increasing drug levels and the risk of sedation or toxicity.

Stimulant herbs like Guarana, Ephedra, Yohimbe, Vacha, and Bala may counteract Clonazepam's calming effects, potentially increasing anxiety or nervous system agitation. Diuretic or purgative herbs such as Senna, Aloe, Dandelion, and Punarnava may disrupt electrolyte balance, heightening the risk of side effects, especially in seizure-prone individuals.

Given Clonazepam's long half-life, strong sedative properties, and potential for dependence, all herbal supplements should be used with caution and under the guidance of a healthcare provider when taken alongside this medication.

Clopidogrel (*Plavix, Iscover*), an antiplatelet medication used to prevent blood clots in conditions such as heart attack, stroke, and peripheral artery disease, can interact with numerous Western and Ayurvedic herbs, especially those that affect blood clotting, liver enzymes, or antioxidant pathways.

Herbs with blood-thinning or antiplatelet properties—including Garlic, Ginger, Ginkgo, Turmeric, Feverfew, and Willow Bark—can amplify the anticoagulant effects of Clopidogrel, increasing the risk of bruising, nosebleeds, gastrointestinal bleeding, or even intracranial hemorrhage. Similarly, Ayurvedic herbs such as Guggulu, Haridra, Arjuna, and Shallaki may have mild to moderate antiplatelet or blood-thinning effects and should be used cautiously in combination.

Clopidogrel is a prodrug that must be converted into its active form by the liver enzyme CYP2C19, making it vulnerable to metabolic interference.

Herbs like St. John's Wort may reduce Clopidogrel's effectiveness by accelerating its metabolism, while Goldenseal, Grapefruit, and in Ayurveda, Licorice, Pippali, and Tulsi may inhibit CYP enzymes and potentially impair activation of the drug, leading to reduced antiplatelet activity and higher risk of clot formation.

Strong antioxidants such as Green Tea, Milk Thistle, and Amalaki may also influence platelet aggregation or hepatic function, though their clinical significance with Clopidogrel remains uncertain.

Because of Clopidogrel's reliance on liver metabolism and its delicate balance between clot prevention and bleeding risk, combining it with herbal supplements—particularly those affecting coagulation or liver enzymes—should be approached with caution and discussed with a healthcare professional.

Codeine (*Tylenol+Codeine, Cheratussin*), an opioid analgesic used for mild to moderate pain and cough suppression, poses significant risks when combined with various Western and Ayurvedic herbs due to its central nervous system depressant effects, metabolic variability, and potential for dependence.

Herbs with sedative or calming properties—including Valerian, Kava, Hops, Skullcap, Passionflower, Chamomile, and Lemon Balm—can enhance codeine's depressant effects on the brain and respiratory system, increasing the risk of excessive drowsiness, confusion, respiratory depression, and in high doses, even coma. Ayurvedic herbs such as Ashwagandha, Tagara, Jatamansi, Shankhapushpi, and Brahmi may similarly intensify these effects, particularly in sensitive individuals. Codeine is metabolized primarily by the liver enzyme CYP2D6, which converts it into its more active form, morphine.

Herbs that affect this pathway—such as Goldenseal, Grapefruit, and in Ayurveda, Licorice, Tulsi, and Pippali—

can either inhibit or accelerate codeine metabolism, leading to reduced pain relief or dangerously high morphine levels, depending on the individual's genetic profile.

Stimulant herbs like Ephedra, Yohimbe, Guarana, and Vacha may counteract codeine's sedative effects and strain the cardiovascular and nervous systems, leading to jitteriness or irregular heart rhythms. Additionally, diuretic or laxative herbs such as Senna, Aloe, and Punarnava could worsen dehydration or electrolyte imbalances when used alongside codeine, especially if constipation or reduced gut motility occurs—a common side effect of opioids.

Because codeine affects both pain perception and respiration and carries a risk of addiction and overdose, combining it with herbal products requires caution and should only be done with the guidance of a knowledgeable healthcare provider.

Cyclobenzaprine (*Flexeril, Amrix, Fexmid*), a centrally acting muscle relaxant structurally related to tricyclic antidepressants, is commonly used to relieve muscle spasms and associated pain but can interact with various Western and Ayurvedic herbs through mechanisms involving sedation, serotonin modulation, and liver metabolism.

Sedative and anxiolytic herbs—such as Valerian, Kava, Skullcap, Hops, Passionflower, Lemon Balm, and Chamomile—can intensify the CNS depressant effects of Cyclobenzaprine, increasing the risk of drowsiness, dizziness, confusion, and impaired coordination. Similarly, Ayurvedic herbs like Ashwagandha, Tagara, Shankhapushpi, Brahmi, and Jatamansi may have additive calming or muscle-relaxing effects that could lead to excessive sedation.

Cyclobenzaprine also carries a mild risk of serotonin syndrome, particularly if combined with serotonergic herbs like St. John's Wort, 5-HTP, SAMe, Turmeric, or Mucuna Pruriens, which may raise serotonin levels and potentially cause agitation, sweating, or tremors.

The drug is metabolized primarily via CYP1A2, so enzyme-modulating herbs such as Goldenseal, Grapefruit, Milk Thistle, and in Ayurveda, Pippali, Tulsi, and Bhumyamalaki may alter its metabolism and either increase side effects or reduce efficacy.

Stimulant herbs like Guarana, Ephedra, Yohimbe, and in Ayurveda, Vacha and Bala, may counteract Cyclobenzaprine's relaxing effects and heighten sympathetic nervous system activity, potentially worsening muscle tension or sleep disturbance. Because of the drug's sedative profile and serotonin-related risks, it is advisable to avoid combining it with herbal supplements unless under professional supervision, particularly when multiple herbs are used concurrently.

Diazepam (*Valium, Valtoco, Diastat, Dizac*), a long-acting benzodiazepine used for anxiety, muscle spasms, seizures, and alcohol withdrawal, is highly susceptible to interactions with both Western and Ayurvedic herbs, especially those with sedative, hypnotic, or hepatic enzyme-modulating effects.

Many calming or nervine herbs—including Valerian, Kava, Skullcap, Hops, Chamomile, Passionflower, and Lemon Balm—can significantly enhance the sedative and depressant effects of Diazepam, increasing the risk of drowsiness, confusion, poor coordination, or respiratory depression.

Ayurvedic herbs such as Ashwagandha, Jatamansi, Tagara, Shankhapushpi, Brahmi, and Mandukaparni may have similar synergistic effects, especially in high or concentrated doses.

Diazepam is metabolized through the cytochrome P450 system, particularly CYP3A4, so herbs like St. John's Wort, Goldenseal, Grapefruit, and in Ayurveda, Tulsi, Pippali, and Bhumyamalaki, may alter its metabolism—either lowering drug levels and efficacy or raising them and increasing side effects.

Stimulant or activating herbs such as Guarana, Ephedra, Yohimbe, and in Ayurveda, Vacha and Bala, may antagonize Diazepam's calming effects and create a tug-of-war in the nervous system, possibly worsening anxiety or tremors. Laxative or diuretic herbs like Senna, Aloe, Dandelion, and Punarnava could contribute to electrolyte disturbances that may heighten sensitivity to Diazepam's central nervous system effects. Because of its long half-life and strong action on GABA receptors, Diazepam should not be combined casually with herbal supplements, especially those that affect sedation or liver function, without careful oversight.

Digoxin (*Lanoxin, Digitek*), a cardiac glycoside used in the management of heart failure and certain arrhythmias, has a narrow therapeutic index and can interact dangerously with numerous Western and Ayurvedic herbs, especially those that affect potassium levels, heart rhythm, or drug metabolism.

Herbs that deplete potassium—such as Licorice, Dandelion (leaf or root in excess), and in Ayurveda, Punarnava and Trivrit—can increase the risk of digoxin toxicity by enhancing its effects on the heart.

Herbs with direct cardiac effects, including Hawthorn, Lily of the Valley, Oleander, and in Ayurveda, Arjuna and Sarpagandha, may either synergize with or oppose digoxin, leading to unpredictable changes in heart rate or rhythm.

Stimulant herbs like Ephedra, Yohimbe, and in Ayurveda, Vacha and Bala, can increase the risk of arrhythmia when combined with digoxin. Certain sedative or nervine herbs such as Valerian, Skullcap, and Jatamansi may interfere with cardiac conduction or mask signs of toxicity like confusion or fatigue.

Digoxin is also affected by P-glycoprotein transport and CYP3A4 enzyme systems, so herbs like St. John's Wort, Goldenseal, Grapefruit, Milk Thistle, and in Ayurveda, Pippali and Tulsi, may alter digoxin blood levels—either reducing its effectiveness or increasing the risk of toxic accumulation.

Importantly, some herbs such as Aloe (in high laxative doses), Cascara Sagrada, and Senna can cause electrolyte imbalances that further heighten toxicity risks. Because symptoms of digoxin toxicity—nausea, visual changes, arrhythmia—can be subtle and life-threatening, combining it with any herbal supplement should be done only with supervision.

Diltiazem (*Cardizem, Cartia XT*), a calcium channel blocker used primarily for hypertension, angina, and certain arrhythmias, can interact with a number of Western and Ayurvedic herbs, particularly those that affect heart rhythm, blood pressure, liver enzymes, or sedation. Herbs with hypotensive properties—such as Hawthorn, Garlic, Motherwort, and in Ayurveda, Arjuna, Ashwagandha, Jatamansi, and Sarpagandha—may amplify the blood pressure-lowering effects of Diltiazem, potentially leading to dizziness, lightheadedness, or fainting. Sedative herbs like Valerian, Skullcap, Passionflower, Lemon Balm, Kava, and in Ayurveda, Tagara, Shankhapushpi, and Brahmi, may enhance the bradycardic (heart-slowing) and CNS-depressant effects of the drug. Diltiazem is metabolized primarily by the cytochrome P450 system, especially CYP3A4, making it vulnerable to interactions with enzyme-modulating herbs. These include potent inhibitors like Grapefruit, Goldenseal, Milk Thistle, and in Ayurveda, Licorice, Tulsi, and Pippali, which can increase Diltiazem levels and the risk of side effects such as edema, bradycardia, or AV block. Herbs with stimulant or sympathomimetic activity—such as Ephedra, Yohimbe, Guarana, and in Ayurveda, Vacha and Bala—can antagonize the therapeutic effects of Diltiazem and may provoke arrhythmias or elevated blood pressure. Additionally, the use of cardiac-active herbs like Digitalis (Foxglove) or potentially toxic Ayurvedic preparations containing Aconite should be strictly avoided, as they may unpredictably affect cardiac conduction. Because of the narrow therapeutic index and cardiovascular implications of Diltiazem, any herbal supplement should be reviewed by a healthcare professional before use.

Doxycycline (*Vibramycin, Doryx*), a broad-spectrum tetracycline antibiotic, may interact with several Western and Ayurvedic herbs in ways that affect its absorption, metabolism, or side effect profile. Herbs high in minerals such as calcium, magnesium, or iron—including Alfalfa, Nettle, Horsetail, and mineral-rich Ayurvedic preparations like Shankha Bhasma and Praval Pishti—can bind to Doxycycline in the gastrointestinal tract and significantly reduce its absorption if taken simultaneously. Tannin-rich herbs such as Triphala and Guduchi may have a similar chelating effect, interfering with bioavailability. Liver-modulating herbs like Goldenseal, Milk Thistle, Licorice, Bhumyamalaki, Tulsi, and Pippali may influence cytochrome P450 enzymes involved in the metabolism of Doxycycline, though the antibiotic is less heavily reliant on hepatic pathways than many others. Immune-modulating herbs such as Echinacea, Astragalus, Ashwagandha, and Amalaki may either complement or counteract the drug's intended therapeutic effects depending on timing and immune context. Finally, herbs known to increase photosensitivity—such as St. John's Wort, Borage, and in Ayurveda, Haridra (Turmeric)—can amplify one of Doxycycline's most common side effects: sun sensitivity. To minimize risk, it is recommended to space the timing of herbal supplements and Doxycycline by several hours, avoid concurrent use of mineral-rich formulations, and consult a qualified practitioner when combining herbs with antibiotic therapy.

Duloxetine (*Cymbalta, Irenka*), a serotonin-norepinephrine reuptake inhibitor (SNRI), shares many potential herb-drug interactions with SSRIs but also adds risks due to its action on both serotonin and norepinephrine. Herbs that may increase serotonin levels, such as St. John's wort, 5-HTP, SAMe, Mucuna pruriens (Kapikacchu) , Jatamansi, Turmeric, and Tagara, can heighten the risk of serotonin syndrome when taken with duloxetine.
Additionally, stimulant or dopaminergic herbs like Yohimbe, Ephedra, Guarana, Cola Nut, Bala, and Vacha may exacerbate duloxetine's noradrenergic effects, potentially leading to increased blood pressure, anxiety, agitation, or insomnia.

Sedative herbs, including Valerian, Kava, Skullcap, Lemon Balm, Lavender, Ashwagandha, Chamomile, Shankhapushpi, Jatamansi, and Tagara, may intensify duloxetine's side effects such as dizziness, fatigue, or confusion.

Several herbs can interfere with the drug's metabolism by affecting cytochrome P450 enzymes, especially CYP1A2 and CYP2D6, which play key roles in processing duloxetine. These include Goldenseal, Grapefruit, Milk Thistle, Licorice, Pippali, Tulsi, and Haritaki, potentially resulting in altered drug levels and reduced therapeutic effect or toxicity.

Herbs with mood-elevating, adaptogenic, or hormonal effects—such as Rhodiola, Shilajit, Dong Quai, and Shatavari—may unpredictably influence emotional stability, particularly in individuals with mood disorders. Given duloxetine's dual mechanism and metabolic profile, it is essential to evaluate herbal supplements carefully before combining them.

Escitalopram (*Lexipro, Cipralex*), an SSRI antidepressant, can interact with a wide range of Western and Ayurvedic herbs beyond the well-known serotonergic agents like Saint John's Wort, 5-HTP, and SAMe. These interactions may increase the risk of serotonin syndrome, excessive sedation, or altered drug metabolism.

Certain herbs, such as Nutmeg, Turmeric, Yohimbe, Mucuna pruriens (Kapikacchu), Jatamansi, and Tagara may enhance serotonergic activity, potentially compounding the effects of escitalopram and contributing to serotonin overload.

Many calming or adaptogenic herbs—including Valerian, Hops, Skullcap, California Poppy, Lemon Balm, Lavender, Jatamansi, Shankhapushpi, Tagara, and Ashwagandha—

may cause additive sedation when used alongside escitalopram.

Others, like Goldenseal, Grapefruit, Nilk Thistle, Licorice, Pippali, Haritaki, and Tulsi, can interfere with liver enzymes such as CYP3A4 or CYP2D6 that metabolize escitalopram, thus affecting its blood concentration and efficacy. Some herbs with stimulating or mood-elevating effects, such as Ephedra, Guarana, Cola Nut, Vacha (Acorus calamus), Bala (Sida cordifolia), and Rhodiola, may provoke overstimulation or mood instability, especially in individuals with underlying anxiety or bipolar tendencies. Finally, herbs with hormonal effects such as Dong Quai and Shatavari may subtly interfere with escitalopram's secondary endocrine influences. For individuals taking SSRIs, caution and professional guidance are advised.

Esomeprazole (*Nexium, Vimovo*), is a proton-pump inhibitor that suppresses gastric acid by blocking the H^+/K^+-ATPase in parietal cells. It is metabolised mainly through CYP2C19 and, to a lesser extent, CYP3A4. Western herbs that can interfere with these pathways or intensify acid-related effects include Saint John's Wort, a strong inducer of both enzymes that may lower esomeprazole blood levels and blunt its acid-suppressive action; Goldenseal and, to a milder degree, Milk Thistle, which inhibit CYP2C19 and could raise esomeprazole exposure and side-effects; Ginkgo biloba and Chamomile, each shown in limited studies to stimulate CYP2C19 activity, potentially reducing drug efficacy; and salicylate-rich plants such as Willow Bark or Meadowsweet, which add gastrointestinal-irritant potential to the acid suppression of esomeprazole, increasing the risk of silent ulcer bleeding.

Mucilage-rich herbs like Slippery Elm, Marshmallow Root and deglycyrrhizinated Licorice do not affect liver enzymes but can physically coat the gastric lining; when taken close to a PPI dose they may slow esomeprazole absorption and delay onset of action, while full-strength (i.e., non-deglycyrrhizinated) Licorice (with glycyrrhizin intact) can raise cortisol and blood pressure, indirectly complicating long-term PPI therapy. Peppermint and Ginger relax the lower esophageal sphincter and speed gastric emptying, which may counteract esomeprazole's benefit in reflux patients, whereas high-dose garlic or turmeric can further inhibit platelet aggregation and slightly raise the risk of gastrointestinal bleeding that is sometimes masked by reduced acid.

In the Ayurvedic materia medica, several dravyas likewise modulate acid balance or hepatic enzymes. Haridra (Turmeric) and its curcuminoids inhibit CYP3A4 and CYP2C19, so regular high-potency extracts can increase plasma esomeprazole levels; at the same time Turmeric's additional antiplatelet and gastric-soothing actions parallel the concerns seen with its Western use. Licorice (Yashtimadhu, Glycyrrhiza glabra) in its whole form potentiates mucus secretion and can delay absorption of concurrently taken medications, while its glycyrrhizin fraction carries the same mineral-corticoid effects noted above. Triphala, rich in Amla's/Amalaki's natural acids and tannins, may lower gastric pH temporarily after ingestion and thus oppose the pH-raising aim of esomeprazole if taken at the same time; taken hours apart, it may exacerbate PPI-related reductions in nutrient absorption by hastening intestinal transit. Kumari (aloe vera) juice is soothing but, in concentrated extracts, can accelerate intestinal motility and interfere with the timing of esomeprazole absorption, and long-term use has been linked to potassium loss that may be clinically relevant in polypharmacy. Guduchi and Tulsi have been reported to mildly induce CYP3A4, suggesting a potential—though usually modest—reduction in esomeprazole exposure, while Shatavari's demulcent saponins can coat the gut lining in a way similar to slippery elm.

When these herbs are combined with esomeprazole, careful spacing of doses and monitoring for reduced efficacy (persistent reflux) or enhanced side-effects (headache, diarrhea, low magnesium) is warranted, and any sustained herbal regimen should be reviewed with a healthcare provider to individualize timing and dose adjustments.

Estradiol (*Estrace, Climara*), is a form of estrogen used in hormone replacement therapy and in the management of menopausal symptoms, menstrual irregularities, and certain hormone-sensitive conditions. Because it is a powerful hormone, herbs—both Western and Ayurvedic—that influence estrogen levels, hormone metabolism, or liver enzyme activity may interact with estradiol. These interactions can either enhance or inhibit its effects, potentially affecting efficacy, side effects, or hormonal balance.

In Western herbal medicine, several herbs are known to have phytoestrogenic properties, meaning they contain plant-based compounds that mimic estrogen. Red Clover and Black Cohosh are two of the most widely used in menopause support. When taken with estradiol, they may increase estrogenic effects, which could intensify symptoms like breast tenderness, bloating, or raise the risk of estrogen-sensitive conditions. Dong Quai, often used in traditional Chinese medicine but also adopted in the West, has mild estrogen-like activity and may also amplify estradiol's hormonal actions. On the other hand, herbs like Saint John's Wort can induce liver enzymes, particularly CYP3A4, which may increase the metabolism of estradiol and lower its levels in the body, potentially reducing its effectiveness. Flaxseed, often consumed for its phytoestrogens and fiber, may also modestly affect estrogen balance and could enhance estradiol's effects when taken regularly.

In Ayurvedic medicine, herbs that influence reproductive and hormonal function may interact with estradiol as well. Shatavari is perhaps the most prominent, widely used to support female reproductive health. It has phytoestrogenic properties and may enhance or modify the effects of estradiol, potentially leading to increased hormonal symptoms if not dosed carefully. Ashoka, another herb used for gynecological health, may also influence hormonal balance and could have additive effects with estradiol. Licorice Root, or Yashtimadhu, can mimic estrogen to some extent and may increase the hormonal load when combined with estradiol, raising the risk of side effects in estrogen-sensitive individuals. Ashwagandha, though primarily an adaptogen, may subtly influence hormonal pathways and stress-related hormone fluctuations, which could affect the body's overall endocrine response when used with estradiol. Guggulu, often used to support detoxification and hormone balance, may affect liver metabolism and influence how estradiol is processed.

Because estradiol therapy requires careful hormonal regulation, any herbs that have estrogenic, anti-estrogenic, or liver-modulating effects should be used cautiously. The combined effects of plant estrogens and pharmaceutical estradiol can lead to hormonal excess or interfere with proper metabolism and clearance of the hormone.

Etanercept (*Enbrel, Erelzi*), is a biologic medication that works by inhibiting tumor necrosis factor-alpha (TNF-α), a key cytokine involved in inflammation. It is commonly used to treat autoimmune conditions such as rheumatoid arthritis, psoriasis, and ankylosing spondylitis. Because etanercept suppresses part of the immune system, the primary concern with herb interactions—both Western and Ayurvedic—involves those that either stimulate or suppress immune function, modulate inflammation, or affect liver metabolism. Herbs that boost immunity or provoke immune activity may reduce the effectiveness of etanercept or worsen autoimmune symptoms, while those with strong anti-inflammatory or immunosuppressive effects may increase the risk of infection when combined with the drug.
In Western herbal medicine, Echinacea is a widely used immune stimulant, often taken to prevent or treat colds. This immune-activating property may theoretically counteract etanercept's immunosuppressive action and could worsen autoimmune symptoms in sensitive individuals. Similarly, Astragalus, another popular herb used to strengthen immune defense, may oppose etanercept's mechanism and is typically not recommended in autoimmune conditions unless closely monitored. On the other hand, Turmeric and its active compound Curcumin have strong anti-inflammatory properties and are sometimes used for joint health. While these may seem to complement etanercept's effects, there is a concern that the combination might increase the risk of suppressing the immune system too much, potentially raising the likelihood of infections.

Other herbs like Cat's Claw and Boswellia (Frankincense) are used for inflammatory conditions but have complex effects on immunity and should be used cautiously with biologic therapies. Saint John's Wort, though not directly related to immunity, induces liver enzymes and can potentially alter the metabolism of other medications, though etanercept is not extensively metabolized in the liver and this interaction is likely minor.

In Ayurvedic medicine, several herbs used for inflammatory and autoimmune conditions may interact with etanercept. Ashwagandha is an adaptogen with both immune-modulating and anti-inflammatory properties. In some individuals, it can stimulate the immune system, which might reduce the drug's effectiveness or increase autoimmune activity, though in others it may have a calming effect on inflammation. Guduchi, (Tinospora cordifolia) is another immunomodulator commonly used in Ayurveda that can enhance white blood cell function and may, therefore, counteract the immunosuppressive effect of etanercept. Licorice, especially in its whole form, has mild immunostimulant properties and should be used with care. Amalaki/Amla, one of the components of Triphala, supports immunity and antioxidant activity, and while mild, may also influence immune function in complex ways. Because etanercept alters immune response, any herb that affects immune or inflammatory pathways can theoretically interact with its action. Some combinations may be helpful, while others could reduce efficacy or increase the risk of adverse effects like infection or autoimmune flare.

Finasteride (*Propecia, Proxcar*), commonly prescribed for benign prostatic hyperplasia and male pattern baldness, has a few very significant herbal interactions. Saw

Palmetto is sometimes used for prostate health and may duplicate some of finasteride's hormonal effects, potentially leading to additive side effects like sexual dysfunction or breast tenderness. Herbs with hormonal activity, like Pygeum or Nettle Root, should be monitored for possible synergy.

Among Western herbs, Licorice root is known to lower testosterone levels and may therefore interact indirectly with finasteride's mechanism. Additionally, hormone-enhancing supplements such as DHEA and Tribulus terrestris might oppose the DHT-lowering action of finasteride, resulting in unpredictable hormonal responses. From the Ayurvedic tradition, several herbs may influence hormonal balance and thus potentially interact with finasteride. Ashwagandha is a well-regarded adaptogen that has been shown to modulate testosterone and DHEA levels. While generally considered balancing, it could affect the hormonal equilibrium when combined with finasteride. Shatavari is known for its estrogenic properties and might subtly counteract androgen suppression, though the interaction would likely be mild. Gokshura, which is the Ayurvedic appellation of Tribulus terrestris, is traditionally used as an aphrodisiac and testosterone booster and may therefore diminish the effectiveness of finasteride's DHT suppression. Kapikacchu, or Mucuna pruriens, contains L-DOPA and is also used to support reproductive health and libido, potentially affecting the hormonal balance finasteride seeks to manage.

Vidarikanda, sometimes referred to as Indian Kudzu, is also used for reproductive strength and may have mild estrogenic or adaptogenic effects that influence hormonal pathways.

In essence, most potential interactions between herbs and finasteride arise from their shared influence on testosterone, DHT, or related enzymes. Because these interactions can either enhance or oppose the effects of finasteride, it's important to consult with a knowledgeable practitioner before combining them, especially if you are using finasteride for a medical condition requiring consistent hormonal regulation.

Fluconazole (*Diflucan, Hixdefrima*), an antifungal used for yeast infections, can interact with herbs that affect liver metabolism. St. John's wort may reduce fluconazole's levels by inducing CYP3A4, risking treatment failure. Conversely, herbs that stress the liver, such as Kava or Comfrey, may increase the risk of hepatotoxicity when taken together. Echinacea is sometimes used to support immune function and may also stimulate liver enzymes, although its interaction with fluconazole is less well-documented and more variable. Milk Thistle is frequently used to protect the liver, but it also affects cytochrome P450 enzymes and could theoretically alter how fluconazole is metabolized, though this interaction is generally mild. Goldenseal contains berberine, which has some antifungal activity of its own and may inhibit CYP3A4, potentially increasing fluconazole levels and enhancing both its effects and side effects.
In Ayurvedic practice, several herbs that influence liver function or have antimicrobial properties may interact with fluconazole. For instance, Turmeric, particularly its active compound Curcumin, has been shown to inhibit certain cytochrome P450 enzymes. This could lead to higher levels of fluconazole in the bloodstream. Similarly, Neem is a potent antimicrobial herb with liver-stimulating properties and may affect drug metabolism when taken in large or concentrated doses. Guduchi, (Tinospora cordifolia), is known for its immunomodulatory and

hepatoprotective effects and could subtly alter the way fluconazole is processed by the body, though this interaction is more theoretical than clinically confirmed. Another consideration is Licorice Root, which has some antifungal activity and also influences liver enzyme function; while generally mild in effect, it could modify how fluconazole behaves in the system.

In summary, herbs that either induce or inhibit liver enzymes, particularly CYP3A4, have the potential to interact with fluconazole by altering its metabolism. This may lead to reduced effectiveness or increased side effects, depending on the direction of the interaction. Anyone using fluconazole regularly or for serious infections should consult a healthcare provider before adding herbal supplements, especially those known to affect liver function or drug metabolism.

Fluoxetine (*Prozac, Sarafem*), an SSRI antidepressant, has well-known risks when combined with serotonergic herbs like Saint John's wort, 5-HTP, or SAMe. The combination can cause serotonin syndrome, a potentially dangerous condition characterized by restlessness, sweating, tremor, and even cardiovascular collapse. Ginseng can add overstimulation or insomnia.

Fluoxetine can potentially interact with a number of other Western and Ayurvedic herbs, particularly those that influence mood, serotonin levels, or hepatic metabolism. Among Western herbs, Kava and Valerian, both used for anxiety and sleep, may interact more on the sedative side, potentially exaggerating central nervous system effects when used alongside fluoxetine.

From the Ayurvedic tradition, herbs that affect the nervous system or mood need to be approached with caution when used with fluoxetine. Ashwagandha is a popular adaptogen known for its calming and strengthening effects on the nervous system. While generally regarded as safe, it may have mild effects on neurotransmitter regulation and could either augment or complicate fluoxetine's action in sensitive individuals. Brahmi, or Bacopa monnieri, is another herb that influences mental clarity and has potential serotonergic activity; when combined with fluoxetine, there is a theoretical risk of excessive serotonergic stimulation. Shankhpushpi, which is often used in Ayurvedic formulas for anxiety, memory, and calmness, may act synergistically with SSRIs, though clinical data on direct interactions is limited. Vacha, or calamus root, is considered a nootropic and nervine in Ayurveda and has stimulating properties that may not be ideal alongside fluoxetine, especially in individuals prone to anxiety or insomnia. Licorice, used widely in both Western and Ayurvedic traditions, may also influence corticosteroid and neurotransmitter levels, and while its interaction with fluoxetine is not well defined, it may affect the drug's metabolism or side effect profile.

In essence, any herb or supplement that influences serotonin levels, mood regulation, or liver enzyme activity carries the potential to interact with fluoxetine. Because the consequences of serotonin overload or altered drug metabolism can be serious, it is strongly recommended that any herbal use alongside fluoxetine be closely supervised by a knowledgeable healthcare provider.

Fluticasone (*Flonase, Advair*), an inhaled corticosteroid for asthma and allergies, generally has few herbal interactions because of its local action in the lungs. However, Licorice, when used chronically in large doses, can raise blood pressure and cause fluid retention, which may compound corticosteroid side effects.

Among Western herbs, Saint John's Wort is important to be aware of. It is a known inducer of CYP3A4 and can increase the metabolism of fluticasone, potentially reducing its effectiveness. Echinacea, often taken for immune support, may also affect liver enzymes and could influence how fluticasone is processed, though this effect is less predictable. Ginseng has immune-modulating properties and may theoretically counteract the immunosuppressive effects of corticosteroids like fluticasone. Similarly, Astragalus, another popular immune-boosting herb, could reduce the efficacy of fluticasone by stimulating immune activity in opposition to the drug's suppressive action. Kava and valerian, while primarily sedative herbs, may impact the central nervous system when fluticasone is taken in high doses or alongside other medications, although interactions here are more speculative.

In Ayurveda, several herbs may interact with fluticasone either by affecting its metabolism or counterbalancing its immunosuppressive effects. Turmeric, especially in concentrated curcumin extracts, can inhibit CYP3A4 and potentially increase levels of fluticasone in the body, which might raise the risk of side effects such as adrenal suppression or oral thrush. Neem has strong anti-inflammatory and antimicrobial actions, but it also stimulates immune function and could theoretically reduce the effectiveness of corticosteroids. Guduchi, or Tinospora cordifolia, is another immunomodulating herb commonly used to build resistance against infections, and like Astragalus, it may counter the immune-dampening effects of fluticasone. Ashwagandha is more adaptogenic and less directly immunostimulating but may subtly influence hormonal balance and the stress-response system in ways that could interact with corticosteroid therapy. Tulsi, or holy basil, also has mild anti-inflammatory and immune-supportive actions and may have overlapping or counter-regulatory effects with fluticasone, especially if used long term or in high doses.

Overall, while fluticasone is primarily a locally acting medication, herbs that modify liver enzyme function or immune activity may interact with it by either enhancing its effects and risks or reducing its intended benefits. Monitoring for both reduced efficacy and increased side effects is important when combining fluticasone with herbal treatments, particularly those that affect detoxification pathways or immune modulation.

Furosemide (*Lasix, Furoscix*), a loop diuretic used for fluid retention and heart failure, can interact with herbs that also have diuretic properties. Dandelion Leaf, Corn Silk, or Juniper Berry can add to diuresis, risking dehydration or electrolyte imbalance. Licorice can promote potassium loss, increasing risk of arrhythmias when combined with furosemide.

Herbs that either intensify diuresis, affect kidney function, alter electrolyte levels, or influence blood pressure may interact with furosemide.

Among Western herbs, Licorice root, especially in non-deglycyrrhizinated form, can lead to potassium loss and sodium retention, which may dangerously compound furosemide's potassium-depleting effect and raise blood pressure. Hawthorn, frequently used for heart health, may lower blood pressure and enhance the effects of furosemide, increasing the risk of hypotension. Uva ursi and Horsetail are additional diuretic herbs that may amplify furosemide's action and increase the risk of renal strain or dehydration.

From the Ayurvedic tradition, Punarnava is a key herb with diuretic properties. It is often used to treat edema and support kidney function, but when taken with furosemide, it could intensify fluid and electrolyte loss. Gokshura, commonly used in urinary tract and kidney support formulas, may also mildly enhance diuresis and interact with the action of furosemide. Triphala, though more commonly known as a digestive and detoxifying formula, may have a mild diuretic effect and alter electrolyte balance with long-term use. Arjuna, an important cardiotonic herb in Ayurveda, may affect blood pressure and interact synergistically with furosemide, potentially intensifying its effects. Similarly, Ashwagandha, while primarily an adaptogen, may influence fluid balance and kidney function indirectly, especially in high doses or when used in combination with other herbs that act on the cardiovascular system.

Because furosemide has a narrow therapeutic window and a strong impact on fluid and electrolyte levels, combining it with herbs that influence these same systems requires caution.

Monitoring blood pressure, kidney function, and electrolytes is especially important when using such combinations, and any herbal use should ideally be discussed with a healthcare provider to avoid additive effects or unexpected complications.

Gabapentin (*Neurontin, Gralise*), prescribed for neuropathic pain and seizures, may have additive sedative effects if combined with herbs like Kava or Valerian, increasing drowsiness and dizziness. Saint John's Wort may theoretically lower gabapentin levels by inducing certain metabolic pathways, though this effect is mild.

Although it is not metabolized by the liver and is excreted unchanged through the kidneys, it still has potential to interact with herbs that affect the central nervous system, especially those with sedative, anxiolytic, or nerve-calming effects.

Among other Western herbs, Passionflower and Lemon Balm, both used for nervous tension and sleep, may have additive effects and increase fatigue or mental slowing when taken alongside gabapentin.

In Ayurvedic medicine, Ashwagandha is one of the most commonly used adaptogens and is often employed for anxiety, fatigue, and nervous system support. It may enhance the calming effects of gabapentin and lead to increased sedation in some individuals. Brahmi, or Bacopa monnieri, is another nervine tonic that improves cognition and reduces anxiety, but when taken with gabapentin, it might increase the sedative or cognitive side effects, especially in sensitive individuals. Shankhpushpi, traditionally used to improve memory and reduce anxiety, also acts on the nervous system and may interact similarly. Tagara, the Ayurvedic counterpart to valerian, has sedative properties and could magnify gabapentin's drowsiness or dizziness. Jyotishmati, a lesser-known herb used for nervous system support, may have unpredictable interactions due to its stimulating and adaptogenic qualities.

Although gabapentin is generally well-tolerated, its combination with herbs that affect the brain or nervous system may lead to increased sedation, dizziness, confusion, or in rare cases, reduced seizure control. Anyone using gabapentin along with herbal supplements should be especially mindful of changes in alertness, coordination, or mood and consult a healthcare provider before combining them, particularly if using multiple herbs with calming or stimulating effects.

Glipizide (*Glucotrol, Glucotrol XL*), an oral diabetes medication, should be used cautiously with herbs that lower blood sugar. Bitter Melon, Gurmar (Gymnema), Fenugreek, and Ginseng all have hypoglycemic effects that can push blood sugar too low if not monitored carefully.

Other herbs potentially compounding glipizide's effects inlcude Cinnamon, commonly used for glycemic control, may also lower blood glucose levels and contribute to blood sugar reductions when combined with glipizide. Licorice Root, while often thought of as benign, may impair blood sugar control in some individuals due to its cortisol-like effects, potentially interfering with glipizide's action. From the Ayurvedic tradition, several herbs are regularly used to manage diabetes and may interact with glipizide. Vijaysar, derived from the Pterocarpus marsupium tree, is traditionally used to lower blood sugar and may enhance the glucose-lowering effects of glipizide. Shilajit, though more often used for energy and metabolic support, may subtly improve glucose utilization and enhance insulin sensitivity, potentially adding to glipizide's effect. Turmeric, particularly in concentrated curcumin form, has been shown to improve insulin function and reduce glucose levels, which could also contribute to hypoglycemia when used alongside glipizide.

In summary, both Western and Ayurvedic herbs that lower blood sugar may have additive effects with glipizide, increasing the risk of dangerously low glucose levels. Anyone using glipizide should approach herbal supplementation with care and consult with a healthcare provider, especially when using herbs known for their antidiabetic properties. Monitoring blood glucose closely is essential when combining such therapies to avoid complications.

Hydrochlorothiazide (*Microzide, Hydrodiuril*), a common thiazide diuretic, may have additive effects with herbal diuretics like Dandelion Leaf or Parsley. Licorice can counteract its blood pressure-lowering effect by causing sodium retention. Herbs that lower potassium can increase risk of arrhythmias when combined with thiazides.

Among other Western herbs, Hawthorn, a herb used for cardiovascular support, can lower blood pressure and may enhance the blood pressure-lowering effects of hydrochlorothiazide, potentially leading to hypotension. Similarly, Juniper Berries and Horsetail, both of which have diuretic properties, can intensify the diuretic action of the drug, increasing the likelihood of dehydration and electrolyte imbalance.

In the Ayurvedic tradition, Punarnava is one of the most prominent diuretic herbs and is often used for conditions involving fluid retention or kidney health. When taken along with hydrochlorothiazide, it can amplify fluid loss and exacerbate potassium depletion. Gokshura, traditionally used to support the urinary system, may have mild diuretic properties and contribute to the overall effect on electrolyte excretion. Arjuna, an important herb for heart health, can support circulation and lower blood pressure, which could strengthen hydrochlorothiazide's hypotensive action and increase the risk of low blood pressure. Triphala, while mainly known as a digestive tonic, has mild detoxifying and diuretic properties that could also enhance the fluid-losing effect of the medication. Ashwagandha, although not a diuretic, may influence blood pressure indirectly through its adaptogenic effects and could potentially affect the drug's blood pressure-lowering action in sensitive individuals.

Hydrocodone (*Vicodin, Norco*), an opioid pain reliever often combined with acetaminophen, carries the same cautions as other opioids. Kava, Valerian, and Passionflower can cause excessive sedation and respiratory depression. Saint John's Wort may lower pain relief by speeding up drug metabolism.
Among other Western herbs, Skullcap, both traditionally used to calm the nerves and promote sleep, may similarly magnify hydrocodone's sedative effects.
In Ayurvedic medicine, several herbs used for calming or pain relief may also interact with hydrocodone. Ashwagandha, while generally mild, is a nervine tonic that can have sedative properties; when combined with an opioid, it could increase drowsiness or impair cognition in some individuals. Tagara, often considered the Ayurvedic equivalent of valerian, has more pronounced sedative effects and may significantly enhance the central nervous system depression caused by hydrocodone. Jatamansi, another calming herb used for anxiety and insomnia, could similarly increase the risk of excessive sedation. Brahmi and Shankhpushpi, which are used to support mental clarity and reduce stress, are generally gentler but may still contribute to central nervous system effects when taken with opioids.
In rare cases, herbs like Opium Poppy itself, which is used in some traditional Ayurvedic and Unani formulas, may dangerously amplify hydrocodone's opioid action and should never be combined.
Because hydrocodone already carries significant risks of dependence, respiratory depression, and cognitive

impairment, combining it with herbs that affect the nervous system must be done with extreme caution. Even herbs considered safe or mild on their own can become dangerous when taken alongside opioids. Anyone taking hydrocodone should avoid sedating herbs unless under medical supervision, and should be especially cautious with any substance that affects mood, sleep, or mental clarity.

Ibuprofen (*Advil, Motrin*), a widely used NSAID for pain and inflammation, can interact with herbs that affect bleeding and the stomach lining. Ginkgo, Garlic, and Ginger can add to bleeding risk. Willow Bark may have additive anti-inflammatory effects but also increase gastrointestinal irritation and ulcer risk.
Western and Ayurvedic herbs that influence inflammation, digestion, blood thinning, or kidney health may interact with ibuprofen in potentially harmful ways.
Turmeric and its active compound Curcumin are frequently used for pain and inflammation and may interact with ibuprofen by increasing the likelihood of gastrointestinal discomfort or bleeding, especially at high doses.
In Ayurvedic medicine, certain herbs commonly used for pain and inflammation may interact with ibuprofen as well. Shallaki, or Boswellia serrata, is an effective anti-inflammatory that acts on leukotriene pathways and may amplify the effects of ibuprofen. While potentially beneficial in some contexts, the combination could increase gastrointestinal irritation or burden the kidneys. Guggulu, a resin used to treat inflammatory conditions and joint pain, also has blood-thinning properties and may elevate the risk of bleeding when combined with NSAIDs. Licorice root, especially in non-deglycyrrhizinated form, can raise blood pressure and cause fluid retention, which might

compound the kidney-related side effects of ibuprofen. Additionally, Punarnava, often used as a diuretic and kidney-supporting herb, may alter the renal elimination of ibuprofen, though data on this interaction is limited. Because ibuprofen can affect the gastrointestinal tract, kidneys, and blood clotting, combining it with herbs that influence similar systems should be done with caution. The risk of stomach ulcers, bleeding, or kidney strain may be heightened when anti-inflammatory or blood-thinning herbs are used concurrently.

Insulin (*Lantus, Humalog*), used for type 1 and type 2 diabetes, Insulin is a vital hormone therapy used to manage blood sugar levels in people with diabetes, particularly type 1 and advanced type 2 diabetes. Because it directly lowers blood glucose, any herb that also affects blood sugar—by increasing insulin sensitivity, enhancing insulin secretion, or independently reducing glucose—can interact with insulin. The primary concern with such interactions is hypoglycemia, a potentially dangerous drop in blood sugar levels. Both Ayurvedic and Western herbs with antidiabetic or metabolic effects can magnify insulin's action and should be used with caution. In Western herbal medicine, several commonly used herbs have known blood sugar-lowering effects. Bitter Melon is one of the most potent, as it has insulin-like properties and may significantly lower blood glucose when taken with insulin, increasing the risk of hypoglycemia. Fenugreek seeds are also widely used for their ability to improve insulin sensitivity and slow carbohydrate absorption; when used with insulin, they can enhance its effect on lowering blood sugar. Gymnema sylvestre, although often classified as an Ayurvedic herb, is also popular in Western herbalism and has strong insulin-enhancing effects, potentially leading to low blood sugar when used together with insulin therapy. Cinnamon, particularly in therapeutic doses, has been shown to support glucose metabolism and may subtly enhance insulin action. Alpha-lipoic acid is another natural supplement that may increase insulin sensitivity and interact with insulin treatment.

In Ayurvedic medicine, several herbs are traditionally used for diabetes management and may interact with insulin in similar ways. Gurmar, (Gymnema), has a long history of use in Ayurveda to suppress sweet taste and regulate blood sugar levels; when used alongside insulin, it can strengthen the hypoglycemic effect. Karela (Bitter Gourd), is another potent glucose-lowering herb often recommended for diabetic individuals, but in combination with insulin, it may require careful monitoring of blood sugar to avoid hypoglycemia. Vijaysar, from the Pterocarpus marsupium tree, is a classical antidiabetic remedy and may also intensify insulin's blood sugar-lowering action. Shilajit, while more often used as a general tonic and metabolic booster, can improve insulin function and subtly affect glucose metabolism. Turmeric, especially in concentrated curcumin form, may enhance insulin sensitivity and reduce inflammation, thus modifying insulin's effect.

Because insulin is a powerful medication with a narrow margin of safety, combining it with herbs that affect blood sugar requires close monitoring. Even natural substances can have strong effects on glucose levels, and their interaction with insulin may lead to dangerously low blood sugar if not adjusted appropriately.

Isosorbide mononitrate (*Imdur, Monoket*), is a nitrate medication used primarily to prevent angina, or chest pain, in people with coronary artery disease. It works by relaxing and dilating blood vessels, which improves blood flow to the heart and reduces its workload. The most significant interactions with herbs - both Western and Ayurvedic - arise from those that also affect blood pressure, circulation, or nitric oxide pathways. Because isosorbide mononitrate can cause a drop in blood pressure and lightheadedness, especially when standing, combining it with herbs that have vasodilating or hypotensive effects can lead to excessive lowering of blood pressure, dizziness, or fainting.

In Western herbal medicine, Hawthorn is widely used for heart health and has mild vasodilating and blood pressure-lowering effects. When taken with isosorbide mononitrate, it may amplify the drug's effect on blood vessels and increase the risk of low blood pressure or faintness. Garlic, especially in higher supplemental doses, also promotes blood vessel relaxation and thinning of the blood, which may enhance the hypotensive effect of the nitrate. Ginkgo biloba improves circulation and has mild blood pressure-lowering properties, which when combined with a nitrate, could increase the risk of dizziness or weakness.

Although not an herb, L-arginine, technically an amino acid, is often used in natural medicine to increase nitric oxide levels and dilate blood vessels, potentially producing an additive effect with isosorbide mononitrate.

Similarly, Cocoa or Dark Chocolate, which contains flavonoids that promote nitric oxide production, may have a modest additive effect, though this is more likely in concentrated forms.

In Ayurvedic medicine, Arjuna is the primary herb used for supporting cardiovascular health. It strengthens the heart muscle and may lower blood pressure slightly. If taken with isosorbide mononitrate, it could modestly increase the risk of hypotension. Ashwagandha, while known more for its adaptogenic and calming properties, can also lower blood pressure in some individuals and may enhance the nitrate's blood vessel–relaxing effect. Tulsi, or Holy Basil, is sometimes used to support circulation and manage stress, and although its effects are usually mild, it could subtly reinforce the action of nitrates in sensitive individuals. Brahmi, used for mental clarity and nervous system support, may reduce vascular resistance and blood pressure in some users. Less commonly, herbs like Jatamansi and Shankhpushpi, used in calming and stress-reducing formulas, may also lower blood pressure slightly and could contribute to overall vascular relaxation. Because isosorbide mononitrate already causes significant vasodilation, combining it with herbs that support circulation or reduce blood pressure should be done cautiously. The cumulative effect may lead to lightheadedness, fainting, or more pronounced drops in blood pressure, especially when changing positions or during physical activity.

Lansoprazole (*Prevacid*), can interact with various Western and Ayurvedic herbs, potentially affecting its absorption, metabolism, or therapeutic effect. In Western herbalism, St. John's Wort (Hypericum perforatum) is a well-known inducer of cytochrome P450 enzymes and may reduce lansoprazole's effectiveness by speeding up its breakdown in the liver.
Similarly, herbs like Goldenseal (Hydrastis canadensis) and Garlic (Allium sativum) can affect liver enzymes and may interfere with lansoprazole's metabolism.
Licorice (Glycyrrhiza glabra), used in both Western and Ayurvedic traditions, may increase stomach mucus and reduce acid, overlapping or potentially enhancing

lansoprazole's effects; however, deglycyrrhizinated Licorice (DGL) is generally considered safer and less likely to cause hypertension or potassium loss.

In Ayurveda, herbs that affect digestive fire (agni) such as Ginger (Zingiber officinale), Black Pepper (Piper nigrum), and Trikatu (a blend of black pepper, long pepper, and ginger) may oppose lansoprazole's suppressive action on gastric acid, potentially diminishing its effectiveness or causing discomfort.

On the other hand, soothing herbs like Amalaki (Emblica officinalis) and Shatavari (Asparagus racemosus) may have synergistic effects with lansoprazole, helping to reduce inflammation and promote mucosal healing.

It is also worth noting that herbs containing high tannin or fiber content, such as Triphala or Psyllium husk, may interfere with lansoprazole's absorption if taken at the same time. Therefore, it is best to separate doses by at least 1–2 hours and consult with a healthcare provider or knowledgeable herbalist before combining herbal treatments with prescription medications like lansoprazole.

Lisinopril (*Prinvil, Zestril*), an ACE inhibitor used to treat high blood pressure and heart failure, can interact with several Western and Ayurvedic herbs, sometimes increasing the risk of side effects such as low blood pressure, high potassium levels, or kidney stress. In Western herbalism, Garlic and Hawthorn are commonly used for cardiovascular support, but when combined with Lisinopril, they may amplify its blood pressure-lowering effects and increase the risk of hypotension. Similarly, Danshen (Salvia Miltiorrhiza), an herb used in Chinese medicine but also found in integrative Western practice, may enhance vasodilation and interact adversely.

Herbs high in potassium or those that spare potassium, such as Nettle Leaf or Dandelion Root, can increase the risk of hyperkalemia when used with Lisinopril.
In Ayurvedic practice, Ashwagandha, Shatavari, and Moringa can also contribute to elevated potassium levels. Gokshura, a mild diuretic and tonic for the urinary tract, might further reduce blood pressure or alter kidney function when used alongside Lisinopril. Herbs with diuretic properties, such as Punarnava, may intensify fluid and electrolyte shifts.
Because Lisinopril can already affect potassium levels and kidney function, combining it with herbs that have similar actions, or that increase potassium retention, requires caution. People using Lisinopril should consult a knowledgeable healthcare provider before starting any herbal supplements to avoid unintended interactions or side effects.

Lorazepam (*Ativan, Loreev XR*), a benzodiazepine used for anxiety, insomnia, and muscle relaxation, can interact with a number of Western and Ayurvedic herbs that affect the central nervous system.
In Western herbalism, herbs such as Valerian, Kava, Passionflower, Skullcap, Hops, and Chamomile have sedative or calming properties and may enhance the effects of Lorazepam, leading to excessive drowsiness, dizziness, or even respiratory depression when taken together. St. John's Wort, although often used for mild depression, can interfere with the metabolism of benzodiazepines and may reduce or unpredictably alter Lorazepam's effectiveness.
In Ayurveda, herbs like Ashwagandha, Jatamansi, Brahmi, Tagara, and Shankhpushpi are commonly used for calming the mind and supporting sleep or mental clarity.

While they may seem like gentle options, combining them with Lorazepam could result in increased sedation or impaired coordination, especially in older adults.

Herbs with adaptogenic or nervine actions may also affect how the nervous system responds to the drug, sometimes masking its effects or prolonging them.

Because both Western and Ayurvedic calming herbs act on similar pathways in the brain, it is important to use caution and avoid simultaneous use without guidance.

Combining Lorazepam with other substances that depress the central nervous system, even if natural, can pose risks to safety, especially when driving, operating machinery, or in individuals with compromised health. Consult a healthcare professional before adding herbs to a regimen that includes Lorazepam.

Losartan (*Cozaar, Hyzaar*), an angiotensin II receptor blocker used to treat high blood pressure and protect kidney function, especially in diabetics, can interact with several Western and Ayurvedic herbs, particularly those that influence blood pressure, potassium levels, or kidney function.

In Western herbalism, Garlic and Hawthorn are commonly used for cardiovascular support and may enhance the blood pressure-lowering effect of Losartan, increasing the risk of hypotension. Herbs like Dandelion and Nettle, especially their leaf preparations, are rich in potassium and may contribute to hyperkalemia when combined with Losartan, which already has a tendency to raise potassium levels. Similarly, Alfalfa and Licorice (when not deglycyrrhizinated) may affect electrolyte balance and blood pressure regulation.

In Ayurvedic medicine, herbs such as Ashwagandha, Arjuna, and Jatamansi, often used to support heart health and reduce stress, may have additive hypotensive effects when used with Losartan. Potassium-rich herbs or tonics such as Moringa and Shatavari can also increase the risk of elevated potassium. Diuretic herbs like Punarnava and Gokshura may further affect fluid and electrolyte levels, especially if the person is also taking a diuretic alongside Losartan.

Because Losartan affects kidney filtration and potassium balance, caution should be used when combining it with herbs that have similar or overlapping actions. Regular monitoring of blood pressure, kidney function, and serum potassium is important, and anyone taking Losartan should consult with a healthcare provider before using herbal supplements.

Metformin (*Glucophage, Glucophage XR*), covered earlier, can interact with a variety of Western and Ayurvedic herbs that influence blood sugar levels, insulin sensitivity, or liver function. In Western herbalism, herbs such as Gymnema, Bitter Melon, Fenugreek, Cinnamon, and Berberine-containing plants are commonly used to help manage blood glucose. When taken alongside Metformin, these herbs may have additive effects, potentially leading to hypoglycemia, especially if not carefully monitored. Milk Thistle, often used to support liver function, could alter how the liver processes Metformin, though evidence on this is still emerging.

In Ayurvedic medicine, several herbs traditionally used to balance blood sugar—such as Gudmar, Karela, Vijaysar, and Neem—can enhance the glucose-lowering effect of Metformin and may increase the risk of blood sugar dropping too low. Turmeric, another commonly used herb, may also amplify Metformin's action by improving insulin sensitivity.

While these herbs may seem beneficial when used for the same condition, combining them without medical supervision can result in blood sugar fluctuations or gastrointestinal side effects.

Additionally, some herbs may influence Metformin's absorption or excretion, complicating its dosage. People taking Metformin should be cautious when introducing herbs that affect metabolism, and should regularly monitor their blood sugar levels, particularly if they are using herbs with known hypoglycemic activity. It is essential to consult a healthcare professional before combining Metformin with herbal remedies to ensure both safety and effectiveness.

Methotrexate (*Trexall, Rheumatrex*), used for cancer and autoimmune diseases, can interact with a number of Western and Ayurvedic herbs, especially those that affect the liver, immune system, or detoxification pathways. In Western herbalism, Echinacea is often used to stimulate the immune system, which may counteract Methotrexate's immunosuppressive effects and reduce its efficacy in autoimmune conditions. Milk Thistle, widely known for its liver-supporting properties, may alter Methotrexate metabolism by affecting liver enzymes, potentially either protecting the liver or interfering with the drug's clearance. St. John's Wort can speed up liver metabolism and may reduce Methotrexate levels in the body, decreasing its effectiveness. Herbs such as Alfalfa and Spirulina, sometimes used as natural supplements, may also stimulate immune activity and are best avoided during Methotrexate treatment. In Ayurvedic medicine, herbs like Ashwagandha, Guduchi, and Amalaki are used to support immunity and detoxification, but they may also modulate immune responses in ways that conflict with Methotrexate's action. Turmeric, while anti-inflammatory, has blood-thinning properties and could increase the risk of gastrointestinal irritation or bleeding, especially when liver stress is present. Additionally, herbs like Neem or Guggulu may have immune-activating effects and should be used with caution. Because Methotrexate is metabolized in the liver and can be toxic at higher levels, combining it with herbs that affect liver function or immune modulation can be risky. Close supervision by a healthcare provider is essential if any herbal supplements are considered while taking Methotrexate.

Methyldopa (*Aldoril, Aldomet*), an older but still-used antihypertensive medication, works by reducing sympathetic nervous system activity and lowering blood pressure. Several Western and Ayurvedic herbs can interact with Methyldopa, either by enhancing its effects or counteracting them. In Western herbalism, herbs such as Hawthorn and Garlic are known for their cardiovascular benefits and may amplify Methyldopa's blood pressure-lowering action, potentially leading to symptoms like dizziness, fainting, or fatigue. Diuretic herbs like Dandelion and Nettle may further reduce blood pressure or alter electrolyte balance, increasing the risk of hypotension. Licorice, especially in its non-deglycyrrhizinated form, can raise blood pressure and counteract Methyldopa's effect, making it a poor combination.
In Ayurveda, similar caution applies to herbs that lower blood pressure, such as Ashwagandha, Arjuna, and Jatamansi, which may strengthen the hypotensive effects of Methyldopa and cause excessive lowering of blood pressure if taken together.
On the other hand, Ayurvedic herbs like Guggulu and certain preparations containing stimulating or warming

spices may interfere with Methyldopa's calming action on the nervous system.

Because Methyldopa can also affect liver function and is known to cause drowsiness or fatigue, combining it with herbs that impact energy, blood pressure, or hepatic metabolism should be done cautiously. Monitoring blood pressure closely and consulting a healthcare provider before using herbal supplements is essential to prevent adverse interactions.

Metoprolol (*Lopressor, Toprol XL*), as noted earlier, is a beta-blocker used to treat high blood pressure, angina, and certain heart rhythm disorders, can interact with various Western and Ayurvedic herbs that influence heart rate, blood pressure, or nervous system function.

In Western herbalism, herbs such as Hawthorn and Garlic are often used to support cardiovascular health but may intensify the blood pressure-lowering effects of Metoprolol, increasing the risk of hypotension, dizziness, or fainting. Other calming herbs like Valerian, Passionflower, and Lemon Balm may compound Metoprolol's effects on heart rate and sedation, potentially leading to excessive drowsiness or bradycardia. St. John's Wort, known for its effects on liver enzymes, may reduce the effectiveness of Metoprolol by increasing its metabolism.

In Ayurveda, herbs such as Arjuna and Ashwagandha are frequently used to support heart function and reduce stress.

While beneficial in some contexts, these herbs may also enhance the action of Metoprolol on the cardiovascular system, resulting in low heart rate or blood pressure. Herbs like Jatamansi and Brahmi, which have calming effects on the nervous system, may also increase sedation when combined with Metoprolol.

Because Metoprolol affects both cardiovascular and nervous system function, combining it with herbs that act on the same systems can result in additive effects or unexpected interactions. It is important to monitor heart rate and blood pressure closely and to consult a qualified healthcare provider before combining Metoprolol with herbal supplements, even those considered natural or gentle.

Montelukast (*Singulair*), a leukotriene receptor antagonist commonly used to manage asthma and allergic rhinitis, generally has fewer herb-drug interactions compared to other medications, but certain Western and Ayurvedic herbs may still influence its effects.

In Western herbalism, St. John's Wort is known to induce liver enzymes that could potentially reduce the effectiveness of Montelukast by increasing its metabolism, although specific data is limited. Herbs with anti-inflammatory or immune-modulating properties, such as Echinacea or Goldenseal, may theoretically counteract Montelukast's mechanism or overstimulate immune responses in individuals with asthma or allergies, possibly increasing the risk of adverse reactions.

In Ayurveda, herbs used to treat respiratory conditions such as Vasaka, Tulsi, Pippali, and Licorice may have complementary effects when taken with Montelukast, potentially helping to reduce inflammation and ease breathing.

However, these same herbs may also increase mucus flow or alter immune activity, which could influence how well Montelukast works in some individuals.

Additionally, adaptogenic herbs like Ashwagandha or Guduchi, though supportive in reducing overall allergic responses and inflammation, could theoretically interact in ways that are not yet fully understood. While no major herb interactions with Montelukast are widely recognized, combining it with herbs that influence the immune system, respiratory function, or liver metabolism should be approached with care, especially in individuals with complex health conditions. It is advisable to consult an experienced herbalist before using herbal remedies alongside Montelukast.

Naproxen (*Aleve, Naprosyn*), an NSAID for pain and inflammation, an interact with a number of Western and Ayurvedic herbs, particularly those that affect bleeding, the gastrointestinal tract, or the kidneys.
In Western herbalism, herbs such as Garlic, Ginger, Ginkgo, and Willow bark can increase the risk of bleeding when taken with Naproxen, especially in people who are already at risk or are using other blood-thinning agents. These herbs may also irritate the stomach lining, compounding Naproxen's known gastrointestinal side effects. St. John's Wort may interfere with Naproxen's metabolism in the liver, potentially altering its effectiveness.
In Ayurveda, herbs like Turmeric and Guggulu, which are used for their anti-inflammatory properties, may enhance the effects of Naproxen but also increase the risk of gastrointestinal irritation or bleeding when used together. Herbs such as Licorice may aggravate stomach lining sensitivity and worsen the risk of ulcers when combined with NSAIDs.
Additionally, diuretic Ayurvedic herbs like Punarnava or Gokshura may increase strain on the kidneys when taken with Naproxen, which already carries a risk of renal stress with long-term use.

Because Naproxen can affect multiple organ systems, combining it with herbs that influence inflammation, blood flow, or digestion requires careful monitoring.
Anyone taking Naproxen regularly should consult a healthcare provider before using herbal supplements to avoid potentially serious interactions.

Nitroglycerin (*Nitrostat, Nitro-Dur, Nitrolingual*), used to treat angina and heart-related chest pain by dilating blood vessels and improving blood flow, can interact with various Western and Ayurvedic herbs that also affect circulation, blood pressure, or vascular tone.
In Western herbalism, Hawthorn is often used for heart health and may amplify the vasodilatory effects of Nitroglycerine, potentially leading to low blood pressure, dizziness, or fainting.
Similarly, Garlic and Ginkgo may enhance blood flow and thin the blood, increasing the risk of hypotension or bleeding, especially when combined with other cardiovascular medications.
St. John's Wort, known to alter liver enzyme activity, may potentially affect how Nitroglycerine is metabolized, although data is limited.
In Ayurveda, herbs such as Arjuna and Ashwagandha are commonly used to strengthen the heart and support circulation. While potentially beneficial, their effects on blood pressure and vascular tone may intensify Nitroglycerine's action, posing risks of lightheadedness or collapse in sensitive individuals.
Other Ayurvedic herbs like Jatamansi, Brahmi, and Gotu Kola, which calm the nervous system and improve cerebral circulation, might also compound Nitroglycerine's effects, especially if used in large doses or alongside other medications for heart conditions.

Because Nitroglycerine has a rapid and potent effect on the cardiovascular system, combining it with herbs that affect vascular function or autonomic regulation should be approached with caution. Consultation with a healthcare provider is important before using any herbs alongside Nitroglycerine to avoid dangerous interactions and ensure safe management of heart conditions.

Olanzapine (*Zyprexa, Lybalvi*), an atypical antipsychotic used primarily for schizophrenia and bipolar disorder, can interact with several Western and Ayurvedic herbs. Among Western herbs, St. John's wort is especially concerning, as it induces liver enzymes that may reduce the effectiveness of olanzapine. Kava and valerian, both used for anxiety or sleep, may amplify the sedative effects of olanzapine, leading to increased drowsiness, confusion, or impaired coordination. Ginkgo may affect blood flow and potentially interact with olanzapine's effects on neurotransmitters, though data is limited.
In Ayurvedic medicine, herbs with strong nervine sedative or psychoactive properties, such as Jatamansi, Tagara (Indian valerian), and Ashwagandha, may increase central nervous system depression when taken with olanzapine, leading to excessive sedation. Brahmi and Shankhpushpi, while generally supportive of cognitive function, may also contribute to excessive drowsiness or interfere with the drug's effects.
Caution should also be used with herbs that influence dopamine or serotonin pathways, as these may interact unpredictably with olanzapine's mechanism of action. Combining any of these herbs with olanzapine should be done only under medical supervision.

Omeprazole *(Prilosec, Zegerid)*, a proton pump inhibitor already discussed, can interact with a number of Western and Ayurvedic herbs.

Among Western herbs, St. John's wort is notable for inducing liver enzymes that may accelerate the metabolism of omeprazole, reducing its therapeutic effect. Ginkgo and garlic, when used regularly, may increase the risk of bleeding, especially if omeprazole contributes to minor gastric irritation or platelet inhibition. Licorice, particularly the non-deglycyrrhizinated form, may interfere with omeprazole's action and contribute to gastrointestinal discomfort or electrolyte imbalance.

In Ayurvedic medicine, herbs like Amla and Haritaki, which support digestion and elimination, may either enhance or conflict with omeprazole's acid-suppressing effects, depending on the individual's constitution. Trikatu—a formula of Black Pepper, Long Pepper, and dry Ginger—can stimulate digestion and potentially reduce the effectiveness of omeprazole by increasing its clearance. Similarly, Chitraka and Musta, which kindle digestive fire, may oppose omeprazole's cooling and acid-reducing actions. Careful monitoring is recommended when combining these herbs with omeprazole, particularly in individuals with sensitive digestion or complex medication regimens.

Ondansetron *(Zopran, Zuplenz)*, a serotonin (5-HT3) receptor antagonist commonly used to prevent nausea and vomiting in chemotherapy, etc., can interact with several Western and Ayurvedic herbs.

Among Western herbs, St. John's Wort is the most significant, as it may reduce ondansetron's effectiveness by inducing liver enzymes that speed up its metabolism.

In addition, combining ondansetron with serotonin-boosting herbs like Griffonia or high doses of ginseng may increase the risk of serotonin syndrome, a rare but serious condition involving agitation, confusion, and elevated heart rate. Kava and valerian, while not serotonergic, may enhance central nervous system sedation when used with ondansetron.

In Ayurvedic practice, herbs such as Ashwagandha and Jatamansi, which have calming effects on the nervous system, may intensify sedation if it occurs as a side effect of ondansetron. Brahmi and Shankhpushpi, though generally safe, may interact subtly with serotonin regulation and should be used with awareness. Herbs that impact liver metabolism, such as Guduchi and Bhumyamalaki, could potentially alter ondansetron's breakdown, though clinical data are limited.

Because ondansetron affects serotonin pathways, any herb that modulates neurotransmitters should be used with caution and preferably under the supervision of a knowledgeable healthcare provider.

Oxycodone (*Oxycontin, Percocet*), as already noted, is a powerful opioid pain medication, can interact with various Western and Ayurvedic herbs that influence the central nervous system, liver metabolism, or respiratory function. Among Western herbs, St. John's Wort may reduce oxycodone's effectiveness by inducing liver enzymes that accelerate its breakdown, while also increasing the risk of withdrawal symptoms or insufficient pain control. Kava, Valerian, Hops, Skullcap, and Passionflower all have sedative properties and may dangerously enhance the sedative and respiratory depressant effects of oxycodone, leading to increased risk of drowsiness, confusion, or even slowed breathing.

In Ayurvedic medicine, herbs such as ashwagandha, Tagara, Jatamansi, and Shankhpushpi have calming or sedative effects that could compound the central nervous system depression caused by oxycodone. Additionally, herbs like Brahmi and Vacha, while supportive of mental function, may interact unpredictably with oxycodone's effects on mood and alertness. Herbs such as Guduchi and Haritaki, which influence liver detoxification, could potentially alter how oxycodone is metabolized, affecting its potency or duration of action.

Because oxycodone carries a high risk of dependence, respiratory depression, and overdose, any herbal combination—especially with sedatives or metabolic inducers—should be undertaken only with medical supervision.

Pantoprazole (*Protonix, Pantoloc*), another proton pump inhibitor, may interact with several Western and Ayurvedic herbs, particularly those affecting liver enzymes, gastrointestinal function, or mineral absorption. Among Western herbs, St. John's Wort is known to induce liver enzymes and may reduce the effectiveness of Pantoprazole by increasing its metabolism. Licorice, especially in its whole root form, may irritate the stomach lining or counteract Pantoprazole's acid-suppressing effects, potentially worsening reflux or ulcers. Ginkgo and Garlic, when taken in high doses, may contribute to a mild increase in bleeding risk, especially with long-term Pantoprazole use, which can subtly impair platelet function.

In the Ayurvedic tradition, Trikatu—a combination of Black Pepper, Long Pepper, and Dry Ginger—may increase the metabolic clearance of Pantoprazole by stimulating liver enzymes and digestion. Herbs like Chitraka and Musta, which ignite digestive fire, may oppose Pantoprazole's acid-reducing action and provoke symptoms in individuals with acid-sensitive conditions. Amla and Haritaki, while generally beneficial for digestion, may alter gastric pH and transit time in ways that either enhance or reduce the absorption of Pantoprazole or other medications taken with it.

As Pantoprazole is usually taken long term, special care should be taken with any herbs that influence stomach acidity, liver function, or drug metabolism.

Paroxetine (*Paxil, Pexeva*), an SSRI antidepressant, can interact significantly with a range of Western and Ayurvedic herbs.

Among Western herbs, St. John's Wort poses the greatest concern, as it also increases serotonin levels and may lead to serotonin syndrome when combined with Paroxetine. This potentially life-threatening condition is marked by agitation, confusion, tremors, and increased heart rate. Other serotonergic herbs such as Griffonia and high doses of Ginseng may also increase the risk of serotonin overload. Kava, Valerian, and Passionflower, while not serotonergic, can intensify sedative effects and contribute to cognitive dulling or fatigue when used with Paroxetine.

In Ayurvedic medicine, herbs like Ashwagandha, Tagara, Jatamansi, and Shankhpushpi have calming or adaptogenic properties that may reinforce Paroxetine's sedative or mood-stabilizing effects, occasionally leading to excessive drowsiness or mental fog in sensitive individuals. Brahmi and Vacha may also influence neurotransmitter levels and interact subtly with SSRIs, although evidence is limited. Additionally, herbs like Guduchi and Bhumyamalaki, which affect liver metabolism, may alter how Paroxetine is processed in the body.

Because Paroxetine strongly influences the serotonin system and carries risks of withdrawal and interaction, combining it with herbal remedies should be approached with caution and under medical guidance.

Phenobarbital (*Luminal, Sezaby*), used for seizure disorders, has a high potential for interaction with both Western and Ayurvedic herbs due to its powerful effects on the central nervous system and liver enzyme induction. Among Western herbs, St. John's Wort is particularly problematic, as it can further induce liver enzymes and accelerate the metabolism of Phenobarbital, potentially reducing its effectiveness and increasing the risk of breakthrough seizures. Herbs with sedative properties such as Kava, Valerian, Skullcap, Passionflower, and Hops may dangerously amplify the sedative and respiratory-depressant effects of Phenobarbital, increasing the risk of excessive drowsiness, slowed breathing, and impaired coordination.

In the Ayurvedic tradition, herbs such as Ashwagandha, Tagara, Jatamansi, and Shankhpushpi have calming and nervine effects that may heighten central nervous system depression when used with Phenobarbital. Brahmi and Vacha, which also affect mental clarity and neurotransmission, may subtly interact with the drug's effects on cognition and mood. Herbs like Guduchi and Bhumyamalaki, known to influence liver function, could further alter the metabolism of Phenobarbital, either enhancing or reducing its blood levels.

Because Phenobarbital has a narrow therapeutic window and a high risk of drug interactions, any use of herbal supplements alongside it should be closely monitored by a healthcare provider familiar with both conventional and herbal medicine.

Phenytoin (*Dilantin, Phenytek*), has a narrow therapeutic window and is highly sensitive to interactions with both Western and Ayurvedic herbs, especially those that affect liver enzymes, central nervous system activity, or calcium metabolism.

Among Western herbs, St. John's Wort is a major concern, as it induces liver enzymes and can significantly reduce the effectiveness of Phenytoin, leading to loss of seizure control. Conversely, herbs like Ginkgo may lower the seizure threshold and increase the risk of convulsions, especially in individuals with epilepsy. Kava, Valerian, and Skullcap can enhance sedative effects when combined with Phenytoin, leading to excessive drowsiness or impaired cognitive function.

In the Ayurvedic system, herbs such as Ashwagandha, Tagara, Jatamansi, and Shankhpushpi, though traditionally used to calm the nervous system and support mental balance, may intensify the sedative or neurocognitive effects of Phenytoin. Vacha, which has stimulating and psychoactive properties, may unpredictably interact with seizure thresholds or cognitive side effects. Additionally, Guduchi and Bhumyamalaki, both of which modulate liver activity, may alter the metabolism of Phenytoin, either increasing toxicity or reducing its levels below the therapeutic range. Given the importance of maintaining stable blood concentrations of Phenytoin, any concurrent use of herbs should be undertaken with great caution and under the guidance of a healthcare professional trained in both conventional and herbal therapies.

Pioglitazone (*Actos, Actoplus Met*), an oral antidiabetic drug used primarily to treat type 2 diabetes by improving insulin sensitivity, may interact with several Western and Ayurvedic herbs, especially those that influence blood sugar levels, liver function, or fluid balance.

Among Western herbs, Bitter Melon, Fenugreek, and Cinnamon can enhance the glucose-lowering effects of Pioglitazone, potentially leading to hypoglycemia if not carefully monitored. St. John's Wort may alter liver enzyme activity and affect the metabolism of Pioglitazone, possibly reducing its efficacy. Ginseng may also increase insulin sensitivity and contribute to a stronger glucose-lowering effect.

In the Ayurvedic tradition, herbs like Gurmar (Gymnema), Meshashringi, and Vijaysar are known for their hypoglycemic properties and may potentiate the effect of Pioglitazone, increasing the risk of low blood sugar. Other herbs such as Neem, Turmeric, and Amla may also lower glucose levels and should be used with caution.

Additionally, herbs like Punarnava and Gokshura, which have diuretic and fluid-modulating effects, may affect the mild fluid-retaining properties of Pioglitazone and increase the risk of edema. Because Pioglitazone is metabolized in the liver, herbs that influence hepatic enzymes—such as Bhumyamalaki or Guduchi—may impact its breakdown and efficacy.

Any herbal use in conjunction with Pioglitazone should be carefully coordinated with a healthcare provider to avoid unpredictable changes in blood glucose or side effects.

Prednisone (*Deltasone, Rayos*), a corticosteroid used to reduce inflammation and suppress the immune system, interacts with a range of Western and Ayurvedic herbs, particularly those that affect immune function, blood sugar levels, electrolyte balance, and liver metabolism.

Among Western herbs, Licorice is particularly significant, as it can intensify the effects of Prednisone by mimicking corticosteroid activity and increasing the risk of side effects such as water retention, high blood pressure, and low potassium.

St. John's Wort may induce liver enzymes and reduce Prednisone's effectiveness. Echinacea and Astragalus, which stimulate the immune system, may counteract Prednisone's immunosuppressive effects and are generally not recommended during corticosteroid therapy. Herbs like Ginseng and Ashwagandha, although adaptogenic, may alter immune and endocrine responses and require caution when used concurrently.

In the Ayurvedic tradition, Ashwagandha and Guduchi, both known for supporting immunity and resilience, may oppose the immune-suppressing actions of Prednisone or influence hormonal regulation. Licorice, also used in Ayurveda, poses the same risks as in Western use, especially when taken in non-deglycyrrhizinated form. Other herbs such as Bhumyamalaki, Amla, and Haritaki, which support liver function and detoxification, may affect the metabolism of Prednisone.

Because Prednisone affects multiple physiological systems, including glucose metabolism, bone health, and electrolyte balance, any herb with overlapping effects must be used cautiously and only under supervision to avoid unintended interactions or complications.

Pregabalin (*Lyrica, Lyrica CR*), a medication used to treat neuropathic pain, anxiety, and seizures, can interact with various Western and Ayurvedic herbs that affect the central nervous system, mood, or sedation.

Among Western herbs, Valerian, Kava, Skullcap, Passionflower, and Hops may enhance the sedative and calming effects of Pregabalin, potentially leading to excessive drowsiness, dizziness, or slowed reflexes. St. John's Wort, while often used for mood support, may interfere with neurotransmitter balance and either reduce the effectiveness of Pregabalin or increase the risk of side effects such as agitation or confusion. Ginkgo, though generally stimulating, has occasionally been associated with increased seizure risk and should be used cautiously in individuals with seizure disorders.

In the Ayurvedic tradition, Ashwagandha, Tagara, Jatamansi, and Shankhpushpi have calming and nervine actions that may intensify Pregabalin's central nervous system effects, leading to increased sedation or cognitive dulling. Brahmi and Vacha, which influence mental clarity and nerve function, may also modulate the response to Pregabalin, though their effects are typically milder. Herbs such as Guduchi and Bhumyamalaki, which support liver function, might influence how Pregabalin is metabolized or cleared from the body, although specific evidence is limited.

Because Pregabalin affects both mood and nervous system activity, concurrent use with any herb that acts on these systems should be approached with caution and under professional guidance.

Propranolol (*Inderal, InderalLA, Innopran XL*), a beta-blocker used to treat high blood pressure, anxiety, and certain heart conditions, may interact with a number of Western and Ayurvedic herbs that influence cardiovascular function, nervous system activity, or blood sugar regulation.

Among Western herbs, Hawthorn is one of the most significant, as it also lowers blood pressure and may amplify the effects of Propranolol, leading to hypotension or bradycardia. Valerian, Passionflower, and Kava have sedative properties that may enhance the calming or fatigue-inducing effects of Propranolol. St. John's Wort can induce liver enzymes and potentially alter the metabolism of the drug, possibly reducing its effectiveness. Ginseng may interact unpredictably by affecting heart rate or blood pressure.

In the Ayurvedic tradition, herbs such as Arjuna and Pushkaramoola, which are cardioprotective and reduce blood pressure, can increase the hypotensive effects of Propranolol. Ashwagandha, Jatamansi, and Tagara, known for their calming and adaptogenic effects, may further reduce heart rate or amplify sedation when taken with Propranolol. Brahmi and Shankhpushpi, while beneficial for anxiety and cognition, may slightly intensify the nervous system effects of the drug.

Additionally, herbs like Guduchi and Bhumyamalaki may alter liver enzyme activity and influence the metabolism of Propranolol. Because of the drug's effects on both the cardiovascular and nervous systems, any herb with overlapping action should be used with caution and ideally under medical supervision.

Quetiapine (*Seroquel, Seroquel XR*), an atypical antipsychotic used to treat schizophrenia, bipolar disorder, and major depressive disorder, can interact with a variety of Western and Ayurvedic herbs that affect the central nervous system, liver metabolism, or neurotransmitter balance.

Among Western herbs, St. John's Wort is especially concerning because it induces liver enzymes that can reduce blood levels of Quetiapine, lowering its effectiveness and increasing the risk of relapse. Sedative herbs such as Valerian, Kava, Hops, Passionflower, and Skullcap may intensify the drowsiness, cognitive dulling, and motor impairment already associated with Quetiapine. Ginkgo may interfere with neurotransmitter activity and has been reported in some cases to increase the risk of agitation or abnormal behavior when used with psychiatric medications.

In Ayurvedic medicine, herbs such as Ashwagandha, Tagara, Jatamansi, and Shankhpushpi, which have calming, sedative, or adaptogenic properties, may compound Quetiapine's sedative effects, leading to excessive sleepiness or mental fog. Brahmi and Vacha, which influence cognitive function and nervous system activity, may subtly interact with the mood-regulating or antipsychotic effects of the drug.

Additionally, liver-supporting herbs such as Guduchi and Bhumyamalaki could potentially alter the metabolism of Quetiapine, affecting its blood levels.

Because Quetiapine acts on multiple neurotransmitter systems and has a wide range of psychiatric effects, combining it with herbs—especially those that sedate, stimulate, or affect liver function—should be done only with medical supervision.

Ranitidine (*Zantac*), previously used for acid reflux but now largely withdrawn in many countries due to safety concerns, may interact with various Western and Ayurvedic herbs that affect digestion, liver function, or nutrient absorption.

Among Western herbs, Licorice in its whole-root form may counteract the acid-reducing effects of Ranitidine and potentially worsen reflux or gastritis symptoms. St. John's

Wort can induce liver enzymes and might alter the metabolism of Ranitidine, although this interaction is considered mild.

Herbs such as Ginger, Peppermint, and Chamomile, commonly used for digestive complaints, may either soothe or aggravate symptoms depending on the individual and their underlying condition.

In the Ayurvedic tradition, herbs like Trikatu—containing Black Pepper, Long Pepper, and Dry Ginger—can stimulate digestion and potentially reduce Ranitidine's effectiveness by increasing stomach acid production. Similarly, Chitraka and Musta, which kindle digestive fire, may oppose the acid-suppressing effects of the drug. Amla, Haritaki, and Bibhitaki, though generally balancing for digestion, can alter gastric pH and may interfere with how Ranitidine is absorbed or functions in the body. Herbs such as Guduchi and Bhumyamalaki, which support liver detoxification, may modestly affect drug metabolism. While Ranitidine has been largely withdrawn in many countries due to safety concerns, individuals who still use it or similar H2 blockers should be cautious when combining them with herbs that stimulate digestion or alter liver function, and consult a knowledgeable practitioner before doing so. (*Zantac* is now formulated with famotidine)

Rivaroxaban (*Xarelto*), a direct oral anticoagulant used to prevent blood clots, stroke, and deep vein thrombosis, can interact with numerous Western and Ayurvedic herbs that influence blood thinning, liver metabolism, or platelet function.

Among Western herbs, Ginkgo, Garlic, Ginger, and Turmeric are especially important, as they possess antiplatelet or anticoagulant properties that may increase the risk of bleeding when taken with Rivaroxaban. St. John's Wort is also a concern because it induces liver enzymes and can reduce the effectiveness of Rivaroxaban, raising the risk of clot formation. Other herbs such as Feverfew and Willow Bark may similarly potentiate anticoagulant effects and should be used with caution.

In Ayurvedic medicine, herbs like Guggulu, Shallaki, and Haridra (Turmeric) have blood-thinning or anti-inflammatory properties that can enhance the anticoagulant action of Rivaroxaban, increasing bleeding risk. Garlic and Ginger, used in both systems, also pose a significant risk when combined with Rivaroxaban. Additionally, liver-acting herbs like Bhumyamalaki and Guduchi may influence the metabolism of the drug, potentially altering its blood levels.

Because Rivaroxaban has a narrow therapeutic window and no specific reversal agent in many settings, combining it with any herb that affects coagulation or liver function should be approached with extreme caution and always under the supervision of a qualified healthcare provider.

Rosuvastatin (*Crestor, Ezallor*), a statin medication used to lower cholesterol and reduce cardiovascular risk, may interact with several Western and Ayurvedic herbs that influence liver metabolism, muscle function, or lipid regulation.

Among Western herbs, St. John's Wort is particularly significant because it induces liver enzymes that may reduce the effectiveness of Rosuvastatin by increasing its clearance from the body. Red Yeast Rice, which contains natural statin-like compounds, can amplify the cholesterol-lowering effect of Rosuvastatin and increase the risk of muscle-related side effects such as myalgia or, in rare cases, rhabdomyolysis. Niacin may also enhance lipid-lowering effects but raise the risk of liver strain or muscle pain.

In the Ayurvedic tradition, herbs such as Guggulu, Arjuna, and Amalaki are commonly used for cardiovascular health and cholesterol regulation and may potentiate the lipid-lowering effects of Rosuvastatin. While generally supportive, they may increase the risk of adverse effects if combined without monitoring. Herbs like Bhumyamalaki and Guduchi, which support liver function and detoxification, could influence how Rosuvastatin is metabolized. Additionally, Ashwagandha and Shankhpushpi, though primarily used for stress and cognitive support, may indirectly affect lipid balance and interact with the medication's overall metabolic effects. Because Rosuvastatin is processed through the liver and has dose-dependent risks, especially for muscle and liver toxicity, combining it with herbs that affect similar pathways should be done cautiously and under professional supervision.

Sertraline (*Zoloft, Lustral*), a selective serotonin reuptake inhibitor (SSRI) commonly prescribed for depression, anxiety, and related mood disorders, can interact with a variety of Western and Ayurvedic herbs that influence neurotransmitter levels, liver metabolism, or nervous system function.

In Western herbalism, the most well-known concern is with St. John's Wort, which also increases serotonin levels and may lead to serotonin syndrome when combined with Sertraline—a potentially dangerous condition marked by confusion, agitation, sweating, tremors, and rapid heart rate. Other calming herbs such as Valerian, Passionflower, Skullcap, and Hops can amplify the sedative effects of

Sertraline, possibly leading to excessive drowsiness or dizziness. Ginkgo may alter serotonin and dopamine activity in the brain and could interfere with the drug's action, while also increasing the risk of bleeding when combined with SSRIs.

In Ayurvedic medicine, herbs like Brahmi, Shankhpushpi, Ashwagandha, and Jatamansi are often used for calming the mind, enhancing cognition, or improving mood. While potentially supportive, they may also intensify Sertraline's effects on mood and sleep, and in some individuals could lead to increased sedation or overstimulation. Additionally, Ayurvedic herbs that influence liver detoxification, such as Guduchi or Turmeric, might alter Sertraline metabolism, though clinical evidence is limited.

Because Sertraline has a narrow therapeutic window and affects brain chemistry, it should not be combined with herbs that alter neurotransmitter levels, central nervous system activity, or liver enzymes without professional guidance. Close supervision by a healthcare provider is strongly recommended to avoid interactions and ensure safety.

Simvastatin (*Zocor, Vytorin*), Simvastatin, a cholesterol-lowering statin drug, is particularly sensitive to interactions with both Western and Ayurvedic herbs that affect liver enzyme activity, lipid metabolism, or muscle integrity. Among Western herbs, St. John's Wort is a major concern because it strongly induces liver enzymes, especially CYP3A4, which metabolizes Simvastatin. This can significantly reduce the drug's effectiveness and increase the risk of cardiovascular events. Red Yeast Rice contains naturally occurring statin-like compounds and may intensify Simvastatin's lipid-lowering effects, thereby increasing the risk of side effects such as muscle pain, weakness, or, in rare cases, rhabdomyolysis. Grapefruit and its extracts, while not herbs, are also notable for inhibiting the same enzyme and increasing Simvastatin levels in the blood, raising the risk of toxicity.

In the Ayurvedic tradition, Guggulu is widely used to reduce cholesterol and may have a synergistic effect with Simvastatin, potentially enhancing benefits but also the risk of adverse effects. Arjuna and Amalaki are often used for cardiovascular health and could potentiate Simvastatin's effects on lipid profiles. Herbs such as Bhumyamalaki, Guduchi, and Kutki, which support liver function, may alter how Simvastatin is processed, either enhancing or diminishing its activity. Additionally, Ashwagandha and Brahmi, although not directly affecting lipid metabolism, may interact subtly with Simvastatin's metabolic or muscular pathways.

Because Simvastatin has a well-known risk of liver enzyme elevation and muscle toxicity, it is essential to use caution when combining it with herbs that influence similar systems and to consult a knowledgeable healthcare provider for safe integration.

Sitagliptin (*Januvia, Janumet*), an oral antidiabetic medication that enhances insulin secretion by inhibiting the DPP-4 enzyme, may interact with various Western and Ayurvedic herbs that affect blood sugar levels, liver function, or pancreatic activity. Among Western herbs, Gymnema, Bitter Melon, Fenugreek, and Cinnamon have well-known hypoglycemic effects and may enhance the glucose-lowering action of Sitagliptin, potentially leading to hypoglycemia, especially when used in combination. Ginseng may also lower blood glucose and contribute to an additive effect. St. John's Wort, by altering liver enzyme activity, could potentially affect Sitagliptin metabolism, although this interaction is not well documented. In Ayurvedic medicine, herbs such as Gudmar, Meshashringi, Vijaysar, and Neem are frequently used for managing type 2 diabetes and may intensify Sitagliptin's blood sugar-lowering effects, requiring careful monitoring. Amalaki, Haridra, and Triphala may also support glucose metabolism but could contribute to variable blood sugar levels when combined with pharmaceutical therapy. Additionally, liver-supportive herbs such as Bhumyamalaki and Guduchi might influence how Sitagliptin is processed in the body, although the clinical impact of these interactions is uncertain.

Because Sitagliptin does not typically cause hypoglycemia on its own but may do so in combination with other agents, adding herbs with similar actions should be approached with caution and regular blood glucose monitoring under professional guidance.

Spironolactone (*Aldactone, CaroSpir*), a potassium-sparing diuretic commonly used to treat conditions like hypertension, heart failure, and hormonal imbalances, may interact with several Western and Ayurvedic herbs that affect electrolyte levels, fluid balance, or hormone regulation.

Among Western herbs, Licorice is particularly notable because in its non-deglycyrrhizinated form, it can lead to sodium retention and potassium loss, potentially counteracting Spironolactone's potassium-sparing effects and increasing the risk of electrolyte imbalance. On the other hand, high-potassium herbs such as Alfalfa and Dandelion leaf may raise potassium levels further when combined with Spironolactone, heightening the risk of hyperkalemia. Horsetail and Juniper, both diuretic herbs, may intensify fluid loss and alter electrolyte levels unpredictably.

In Ayurvedic medicine, Punarnava is a strong diuretic and may amplify the fluid-reducing effects of Spironolactone, increasing the risk of dehydration or hypotension. Herbs like Gokshura and Varuna, which also support urinary health, could have additive diuretic effects. Additionally, Ashoka, Shatavari, and other hormone-modulating herbs may interact with Spironolactone's anti-androgenic activity, potentially enhancing or opposing its hormonal effects depending on the context. Herbs such as Amalaki and Bhumyamalaki, known for supporting kidney and liver function, may also influence the metabolism or clearance of Spironolactone.

Because of the drug's potential to affect electrolyte balance and hormone pathways, combining it with herbs that act on similar systems should be done cautiously and under the supervision of a qualified practitioner.

Sumatriptan (*Imitrex*), a medication used to relieve migraine headaches by stimulating serotonin (5-HT1) receptors and narrowing blood vessels in the brain, may interact with several Western and Ayurvedic herbs that influence serotonin levels, vascular tone, or nervous system activity.

Among Western herbs, St. John's Wort is the most significant, as it can increase serotonin levels and may heighten the risk of serotonin syndrome when combined with Sumatriptan. This potentially serious condition can present with symptoms such as confusion, agitation, muscle rigidity, and rapid heart rate. Other herbs like Ginseng and possibly 5-HTP or Griffonia (which are often classified as supplements but have herbal origins) may also contribute to excess serotonergic activity. Additionally, sedative herbs such as Valerian, Kava, and Skullcap may enhance drowsiness or dizziness associated with Sumatriptan.

In the Ayurvedic tradition, herbs like Ashwagandha, Jatamansi, Tagara, and Shankhpushpi, which have calming effects on the nervous system, may increase central nervous system depression when used with Sumatriptan, especially in sensitive individuals. Brahmi and Vacha, which influence mental clarity and neurotransmission, may subtly interact with Sumatriptan's effects on the brain's serotonin system. Herbs like Amalaki or Haritaki, although not directly serotonergic, may influence overall vascular tone and digestion, which can affect migraine patterns and responses to treatment. Because Sumatriptan acts strongly on both blood vessels and neurotransmitters, combining it with herbs that influence serotonin or cerebral circulation should be done with caution and only under professional supervision.

Tamoxifen (*Nolvadex*), a selective estrogen receptor modulator used primarily in the treatment and prevention of estrogen receptor–positive breast cancer, can interact with several Western and Ayurvedic herbs that influence hormone levels, liver metabolism, or antioxidant pathways. Among Western herbs, St. John's Wort is the most problematic, as it induces liver enzymes—particularly CYP3A4 and CYP2D6—which can significantly reduce the effectiveness of Tamoxifen by interfering with its conversion into active metabolites. Red Clover, Black Cohosh, and Dong Quai, all of which have phyto-estrogenic properties, may counteract or unpredictably influence Tamoxifen's estrogen-modulating effects, posing potential risks for women with hormone-sensitive cancers. Flaxseed, though generally considered safe, contains lignans that act as weak phytoestrogens and should be used cautiously.

In the Ayurvedic tradition, herbs such as Shatavari and Licorice, which have estrogen-like activity, may also interfere with Tamoxifen's action and should typically be avoided in estrogen receptor–positive conditions. Ashoka and Vidari are additional Ayurvedic herbs with potential hormonal effects that are problematic. On the other hand, herbs like Guduchi, Amalaki, and Turmeric may offer antioxidant and anti-inflammatory support, but high doses could still influence liver metabolism or interact with Tamoxifen's pharmacokinetics.

Because Tamoxifen's effectiveness relies on precise hormonal and metabolic activity, any herbs that affect estrogenic pathways or liver enzyme activity should be used only with the guidance of a healthcare provider experienced in both oncology and herbal medicine.

Tamsulosin (*Flomax, Jalyn*), an alpha-blocker used to treat symptoms of benign prostatic hyperplasia by relaxing the muscles in the prostate and bladder neck, may interact with several Western and Ayurvedic herbs that influence blood pressure, smooth muscle tone, or hormonal balance.

Among Western herbs, Saw Palmetto is the most commonly associated with prostate health and may have additive effects with Tamsulosin, potentially enhancing symptom relief but also increasing the risk of side effects such as dizziness or low blood pressure. Other herbs such as Nettle root and Pygeum may also affect the same pathways and lead to cumulative effects. Additionally, herbs with vasodilatory or hypotensive properties, such as Hawthorn, Garlic, and Ginseng, can amplify Tamsulosin's blood pressure-lowering effects, leading to lightheadedness or fainting, especially when standing up. In the Ayurvedic tradition, herbs like Gokshura and Varuna, often used for urinary tract and prostate support, may have similar synergistic effects with Tamsulosin, affecting urine flow and vascular tone.

Ashwagandha and Shatavari, known for their adaptogenic and hormonal balancing properties, may also subtly influence the therapeutic effect or side effect profile of Tamsulosin, particularly in men with underlying hormonal imbalances. Herbs like Punarnava, which has diuretic and circulatory effects, could contribute to fluctuations in blood pressure when combined with Tamsulosin.

Because this medication evokes orthostatic hypotension, combining it with herbs that affect cardiovascular or urogenital function should be done with caution and under professional supervision.

Terazosin (*Hytrin*), an alpha-adrenergic blocker prescribed for benign prostatic hyperplasia and sometimes for hypertension, can interact with several Western and Ayurvedic herbs that influence vascular tone, blood pressure, urinary function, or hormonal activity.

Among Western herbs, Saw Palmetto is commonly used for prostate health and may enhance the therapeutic effect of Terazosin, but it may also increase the risk of dizziness or hypotension, particularly postural or orthostatic hypotension. Hawthorn, Garlic, Ginseng, and Valerian can lower blood pressure or cause vasodilation, which when combined with Terazosin may lead to excessive lowering of blood pressure, fatigue, or fainting.

In the Ayurvedic tradition, Gokshura and Varuna, both used to support prostate and urinary tract function, may act synergistically with Terazosin to improve urinary flow but also increase the risk of vascular side effects such as lightheadedness or dizziness. Punarnava, a mild diuretic and circulatory stimulant, may amplify Terazosin's blood pressure-lowering effect. Herbs like Ashwagandha and Shatavari, though more subtle in their action, may influence the hormonal or adaptogenic landscape in ways that modify Terazosin's effects in sensitive individuals. Additionally, Rasna and Bala, often used for neuromuscular and circulatory support, may interact with the drug's impact on smooth muscle tone.

Because Terazosin relaxes blood vessels and bladder neck muscles, combining it with herbs that affect similar pathways should be approached cautiously and under the supervision of a qualified healthcare provider.

Topiramate (*Topamax, Qudexy XR*), an anticonvulsant used for epilepsy, migraine prevention, and occasionally for mood disorders or weight loss, can interact with a variety of Western and Ayurvedic herbs that influence the nervous system, electrolyte balance, liver metabolism, or cognitive function.

Among Western herbs, Valerian, Kava, Skullcap, Passionflower, and Hops may increase the sedative effects of Topiramate, leading to enhanced drowsiness, confusion, or impaired coordination. St. John's Wort may lower Topiramate levels by inducing liver enzymes, potentially reducing its effectiveness in seizure control or mood stabilization. Ginkgo is another herb to use with caution, as it may reduce seizure threshold and interfere with the drug's anticonvulsant action.

In Ayurvedic practice, herbs such as Ashwagandha, Jatamansi, Tagara, and Shankhpushpi, which calm the nervous system and promote mental clarity, may intensify the sedative or cognitive effects of Topiramate, particularly in individuals who are sensitive to its side effects. Vacha and Brahmi, known for their influence on memory and cognition, may also interact unpredictably with Topiramate's effects on mental function.

In addition, herbs like Punarnava and Gokshura, which can affect fluid and electrolyte balance, may complicate Topiramate's tendency to cause dehydration or changes in bicarbonate levels.

Because Topiramate affects multiple systems, including neural excitation, renal function, and cognition, any herb that acts on similar pathways should be used cautiously and under close medical guidance.

Tramadol (*Ultram, ConZip*), a centrally acting opioid analgesic used to treat moderate to moderately severe pain, has a complex mechanism involving both opioid receptor activity and serotonin-norepinephrine reuptake inhibition, making it particularly susceptible to interactions with both Western and Ayurvedic herbs that affect neurotransmitters, sedation, or liver metabolism.

Among Western herbs, St. John's Wort is the most concerning, as it can both reduce the effectiveness of Tramadol through enzyme induction and increase the risk of serotonin syndrome due to its serotonergic activity. Other herbs such as Valerian, Kava, Passionflower, Hops, and Skullcap can enhance Tramadol's sedative effects, leading to excessive drowsiness, dizziness, or respiratory depression. Herbs like Ginseng and 5-HTP may also heighten serotonergic activity, increasing the risk of agitation, confusion, or serotonin syndrome, especially at higher doses.

In the Ayurvedic tradition, herbs such as Ashwagandha, Jatamansi, Tagara, and Shankhpushpi, which calm the nervous system, may amplify Tramadol's sedative and central nervous system effects. Brahmi and Vacha, which affect mental alertness and neurotransmitter function, could interact unpredictably with Tramadol's dual action on pain and mood. Liver-supporting herbs such as Guduchi and Bhumyamalaki might alter the drug's metabolism, potentially affecting its potency or duration of action. Because Tramadol carries a risk of dependence, sedation, and serotonin-related side effects, combining it with herbs that influence mood, sedation, or metabolic pathways should be done only under professional supervision.

Trazodone (*Desyrel, Oleptro*), an antidepressant often prescribed for insomnia, anxiety, and major depressive disorder, affects serotonin levels and can cause sedation, making it prone to interactions with both Western and Ayurvedic herbs that influence neurotransmitter activity, sedation, or liver metabolism.

Among Western herbs, St. John's Wort is particularly significant because it also increases serotonin and may raise the risk of serotonin syndrome when combined with Trazodone. This condition can lead to symptoms such as agitation, confusion, tremors, and elevated heart rate. Other herbs like Ginseng and 5-HTP may also contribute to excess serotonergic activity. Sedative herbs including Valerian, Kava, Hops, Skullcap, and Passionflower can amplify Trazodone's sedative effects, increasing the risk of drowsiness, impaired cognition, or slowed reflexes.

In the Ayurvedic tradition, herbs such as Ashwagandha, Tagara, Jatamansi, and Shankhpushpi, known for their calming and nervine properties, may intensify Trazodone's sedating effects and contribute to mental fog or excessive sleepiness in sensitive individuals. Brahmi and Vacha, which modulate nervous system function and cognition, could interact with Trazodone's effects on mood and alertness. Additionally, herbs like Guduchi and Bhumyamalaki that support liver detoxification may influence the metabolism of Trazodone, potentially altering its blood levels and therapeutic response.

Because Trazodone acts on serotonin and has notable sedative properties, it should not be combined with herbs that similarly affect these systems without careful monitoring by a healthcare provider experienced in both pharmacology and herbal medicine.

Triamterene (*Dyrenium, Dyazide*), a potassium-sparing diuretic often used in combination with other medications to treat hypertension or fluid retention, can interact with several Western and Ayurvedic herbs that affect electrolyte balance, fluid metabolism, or kidney function. Among Western herbs, Dandelion leaf and Alfalfa may contribute to elevated potassium levels, especially when taken alongside Triamterene, increasing the risk of hyperkalemia, which can lead to dangerous cardiac symptoms. Licorice, particularly in its whole-root form, may oppose Triamterene's potassium-sparing effects by promoting sodium retention and potassium loss, potentially destabilizing electrolyte levels. Horsetail and Juniper, both traditionally used as diuretics, could enhance fluid loss and further strain kidney function, especially if used long term.

In the Ayurvedic tradition, Punarnava is a powerful diuretic and may amplify the fluid-eliminating effects of Triamterene, possibly leading to dehydration or shifts in sodium and potassium balance. Gokshura and Varuna, commonly used for urinary and kidney support, may also interact with the drug's renal effects, enhancing diuresis or influencing electrolyte excretion. Herbs like Amalaki, Bhumyamalaki, and Guduchi, which support liver and kidney function, could subtly alter how Triamterene is processed or excreted, although specific data are limited. Because Triamterene affects potassium and kidney function, combining it with herbs that influence similar physiological systems requires careful attention to electrolyte monitoring and hydration status, ideally under the supervision of a qualified healthcare practitioner.

Valacyclovir (*Valtrex*), Valacyclovir, an antiviral medication used to treat herpes simplex, shingles, and other viral infections, is generally well tolerated and has fewer herb-drug interactions than many other medications, but certain Western and Ayurvedic herbs may still influence its safety or effectiveness.
Among Western herbs, Echinacea is sometimes used for immune support during viral infections, but it may stimulate immune activity in unpredictable ways and alter the natural course of infection or inflammation, especially in autoimmune-prone individuals. St. John's Wort, known to induce liver enzymes, may potentially affect the metabolism of Valacyclovir, although this effect is likely minor since the drug is primarily eliminated by the kidneys. Herbs with known nephrotoxic effects, such as Aristolochia or excessive doses of Juniper or Horsetail, could pose a risk when combined with Valacyclovir, which can occasionally affect kidney function at high doses or in dehydrated individuals.
In the Ayurvedic tradition, herbs like Punarnava and Gokshura, which support urinary and kidney health, may

be beneficial if used appropriately, but overuse could amplify diuretic effects and strain hydration status, potentially stressing renal elimination of Valacyclovir. Herbs such as Guduchi, Amalaki, and Haritaki, which support immune response and detoxification, are often used in cases of recurrent infections and are generally considered safe, though they may subtly alter the body's response to viral therapy.

Because Valacyclovir depends on kidney clearance, the most significant risk with herb combinations lies in those that affect renal function, hydration, or immune modulation, and these should be monitored in consultation with a healthcare provider.

Valsartan (*Diovan, Entresto*), an angiotensin II receptor blocker (ARB) used to treat high blood pressure and heart failure, may interact with several Western and Ayurvedic herbs that influence blood pressure, potassium levels, kidney function, or vascular tone.

Among Western herbs, Hawthorn is commonly used to support cardiovascular health and may have additive blood pressure–lowering effects when combined with Valsartan, increasing the risk of hypotension, dizziness, or fainting. Garlic and Ginseng may also potentiate the antihypertensive effects of Valsartan, while high-potassium herbs such as Alfalfa and Dandelion leaf could contribute to hyperkalemia, a known risk when taking Valsartan. Licorice in its whole-root form may counteract the antihypertensive effects by promoting sodium retention and potassium loss, which may create an unpredictable electrolyte imbalance.

In the Ayurvedic tradition, herbs like Arjuna and Pushkaramoola, known for their cardioprotective properties, may reinforce the therapeutic effects of

Valsartan but also raise the risk of blood pressure dropping too low. Punarnava and Gokshura, which act as diuretics and support kidney function, may influence fluid and electrolyte balance, further complicating Valsartan's renal effects. Herbs such as Amalaki, Guduchi, and Bhumyamalaki, often used to support liver and kidney function, are generally safe but may subtly alter how the drug is processed or cleared.

Because Valsartan affects blood pressure regulation and potassium retention, any herb that impacts these systems should be used with caution and under medical supervision to avoid excessive hypotension or electrolyte disturbances.

Venlafaxine (*Effexor, Effexor XR*), a serotonin-norepinephrine reuptake inhibitor (SNRI) used to treat depression, anxiety, and certain mood disorders, can interact with a number of Western and Ayurvedic herbs that influence neurotransmitter activity, sedation, or liver metabolism.

Among Western herbs, St. John's Wort is particularly concerning, as it increases serotonin levels and may lead to serotonin syndrome when combined with Venlafaxine. This potentially dangerous condition may present with agitation, tremors, sweating, and confusion. Ginseng, 5-HTP, and Griffonia may also increase serotonergic activity and should be used with caution.

Sedative herbs such as Valerian, Kava, Passionflower, Skullcap, and Hops may intensify drowsiness, dizziness, or cognitive slowing, especially in sensitive individuals.

In Ayurvedic practice, herbs such as Ashwagandha, Jatamansi, Tagara, and Shankhpushpi, which calm the nervous system, may enhance the sedative effects of Venlafaxine, potentially leading to excessive fatigue or mental cloudiness. Brahmi and Vacha, known for their cognitive-enhancing effects, may interact more subtly with Venlafaxine's modulation of mood and mental function. Additionally, herbs such as Guduchi and Bhumyamalaki, which support liver detoxification, might influence the metabolism of Venlafaxine, potentially altering its blood levels.

Because Venlafaxine acts strongly on neurotransmitters and can affect blood pressure, nervous system tone, and alertness, combining it with herbs that have overlapping or opposing actions should be done only with close monitoring by a healthcare provider experienced in both pharmacology and herbal medicine.

Verapamil (*Calan, Verelan*), a calcium channel blocker used to treat high blood pressure, angina, and certain types of arrhythmias, can interact with a number of Western and Ayurvedic herbs that influence cardiovascular function, blood pressure, heart rhythm, or liver metabolism.

Among Western herbs, Hawthorn is particularly important, as it can have additive effects on the heart and vascular system, potentially enhancing Verapamil's ability to lower blood pressure and slow heart rate, but also increasing the risk of hypotension or bradycardia. Garlic and Ginseng may also lower blood pressure and could intensify Verapamil's effects, while Licorice, especially in its whole-root form, may counteract Verapamil by promoting fluid retention and elevating blood pressure. St. John's Wort may reduce Verapamil's effectiveness by inducing liver enzymes that speed up its metabolism.

In the Ayurvedic tradition, herbs such as Arjuna and Pushkaramoola, used to strengthen the heart and regulate blood pressure, may act synergistically with Verapamil, potentially leading to overly low blood pressure or heart rate. Punarnava and Gokshura, with diuretic and renal-supportive properties, may also contribute to shifts in blood pressure and electrolyte balance when used alongside Verapamil. Herbs like Ashwagandha, which helps calm the nervous system, may enhance Verapamil's relaxing effects, while liver-supportive herbs like Guduchi and Bhumyamalaki might influence how the drug is metabolized.

Because Verapamil affects both cardiac rhythm and vascular tone, herbs that overlap with these actions should be used with caution to avoid cardiovascular complications.

Warfarin (*Coumadin, Jantoven*), is one of the most interaction-prone drugs. A widely used anticoagulant, it is prescribed to prevent blood clots, stroke, and heart attacks and is highly sensitive to interactions with both Western and Ayurvedic herbs, particularly those that affect blood clotting, liver metabolism, or vitamin K activity.

Among Western herbs, several are known to increase the risk of bleeding when taken with Warfarin, including Ginkgo, Garlic, Ginger, Turmeric, Feverfew, and Willow Bark. These herbs possess antiplatelet or anticoagulant properties and can dangerously enhance Warfarin's blood-thinning effect. St. John's Wort is also significant because it induces liver enzymes that can reduce Warfarin's effectiveness, increasing the risk of clot formation. On the other hand, Green Tea and Alfalfa are high in vitamin K and may interfere with Warfarin's anticoagulant action, making it less effective.

In the Ayurvedic tradition, herbs such as Guggulu, Haridra (Turmeric), Shallaki, and Neem have blood-thinning or anti-inflammatory effects that may potentiate Warfarin's activity and increase bleeding risk. Garlic and Ginger, used extensively in both Ayurvedic and Western traditions, are especially risky when combined with Warfarin. Additionally, liver-supporting herbs like Guduchi and Bhumyamalaki could alter how Warfarin is metabolized, affecting its blood concentration.

Because Warfarin has a narrow therapeutic window and is influenced by many dietary and metabolic factors, combining it with herbs that affect coagulation, liver enzymes, or vitamin K status should only be done with close medical supervision and regular monitoring of INR levels.

Zolpidem (*Ambien, Ambien CR*), a sedative-hypnotic medication prescribed for short-term treatment of insomnia, acts on GABA receptors in the brain to promote sleep and relaxation. It can interact with a range of Western and Ayurvedic herbs that influence central nervous system activity, especially those with sedative, anxiolytic, or cognitive effects.

Among Western herbs, Valerian, Kava, Passionflower, Skullcap, Hops, and Chamomile may all enhance the sedative effects of Zolpidem, increasing the risk of excessive drowsiness, dizziness, impaired coordination, or even respiratory depression in sensitive individuals. St. John's Wort may reduce the effectiveness of Zolpidem by inducing liver enzymes that increase its metabolism, but it can also unpredictably affect mood and neurotransmitter balance.

In the Ayurvedic tradition, herbs such as Ashwagandha, Tagara, Jatamansi, and Shankhpushpi are often used to calm the mind and support sleep, but when taken alongside Zolpidem, they may intensify sedation and prolong its effects. Brahmi and Vacha, known for enhancing mental clarity, may interact more subtly with Zolpidem's cognitive effects, possibly increasing confusion or grogginess in the morning. While these herbs are generally safe when used individually, combining them with Zolpidem can lead to amplified central nervous system depression.

For this reason, any use of herbal supplements alongside Zolpidem should be closely monitored by a healthcare provider to prevent adverse effects or dependence.

Zonisamide (*Zonegran*), an anticonvulsant used primarily to treat seizures and sometimes prescribed off-label for mood stabilization or weight loss, can interact with various Western and Ayurvedic herbs that influence neurological function, liver metabolism, hydration status, or electrolyte balance.

Among Western herbs, St. John's Wort is a key concern because it induces liver enzymes that may accelerate the metabolism of Zonisamide, potentially reducing its effectiveness in seizure control. Ginkgo should also be used with caution, as it may lower the seizure threshold and increase the risk of breakthrough seizures. Sedative herbs such as Valerian, Kava, Skullcap, Passionflower, and Hops may intensify central nervous system depression when combined with Zonisamide, resulting in excessive drowsiness, confusion, or impaired coordination. Additionally, herbs like Horsetail and Dandelion leaf, which have diuretic properties, could contribute to electrolyte imbalances or dehydration, worsening known side effects of Zonisamide such as kidney stones or metabolic acidosis.

In the Ayurvedic tradition, herbs like Ashwagandha, Jatamansi, Tagara, and Shankhpushpi, which have calming and nervine properties, may enhance the sedative effects of Zonisamide or alter its cognitive impact. Vacha and Brahmi, known to influence memory and neurological tone, might interact unpredictably with Zonisamide's effects on the brain. Diuretic and renal-supportive herbs such as Punarnava and Gokshura should also be used cautiously, as they may contribute to dehydration or kidney strain.

Because Zonisamide affects both neurological and renal function, combining it with herbs that act on similar systems requires careful monitoring and should only be done under careful monitoring and guidance.

Ziprasidone (*Geodon*), an atypical antipsychotic used to treat schizophrenia and bipolar disorder, works primarily by modulating dopamine and serotonin receptors, and carries potential risks such as sedation, QT interval prolongation, and metabolic disturbances.

It can interact with a variety of Western and Ayurvedic herbs that influence neurotransmitters, sedation, cardiac function, or liver metabolism.

Among Western herbs, St. John's Wort is particularly concerning because it can induce liver enzymes and reduce the blood levels of Ziprasidone, potentially diminishing its antipsychotic efficacy. Furthermore, its serotonergic action may increase the risk of serotonin syndrome when combined with Ziprasidone. Sedative herbs such as Valerian, Kava, Skullcap, Hops, and Passionflower may amplify the sedative and cognitive-dulling effects of Ziprasidone, increasing the risk of excessive drowsiness, poor coordination, or mental fog. Ginkgo should be used cautiously as it may influence neurotransmitter activity and has occasionally been associated with seizure risk.

In the Ayurvedic tradition, calming and adaptogenic herbs like Ashwagandha, Jatamansi, Tagara, and Shankhpushpi may increase the sedative load when taken with Ziprasidone, especially in individuals sensitive to central nervous system depression. Brahmi and Vacha, which modulate mental clarity and cognitive function, may interact with Ziprasidone's effects on mood, perception, and alertness. Additionally, herbs like Guduchi and Bhumyamalaki that support liver function could alter the metabolism of Ziprasidone, though data are limited. Given Ziprasidone's potential effects on heart rhythm and the nervous system, any combination with herbs—especially those that affect serotonin, dopamine, or cardiac conduction—should be approached with caution and under medical supervision.

Zoledronic acid (*Reclast, Zometa*), a bisphosphonate used to treat osteoporosis, bone metastases, and high blood calcium levels, acts by inhibiting bone resorption and can have effects on calcium metabolism, kidney function, and inflammatory pathways.
Although it is not extensively metabolized by the liver, it can interact with certain Western and Ayurvedic herbs that influence calcium balance, renal function, or inflammation. Among Western herbs, high-dose or long-term use of Diuretic herbs such as Dandelion leaf, Horsetail, or Juniper may contribute to fluid and electrolyte imbalances, particularly calcium and magnesium loss, which can increase the risk of side effects from Zoledronic acid such as muscle cramps or hypocalcemia. Licorice, especially in its whole-root form, may worsen fluid retention or elevate blood pressure, complicating treatment in sensitive individuals. Anti-inflammatory herbs such as Turmeric or Willow Bark may have overlapping effects with Zoledronic

acid on inflammatory bone processes, although the interaction is generally mild.

In the Ayurvedic tradition, herbs like Punarnava and Gokshura, which act as diuretics and support kidney function, may need to be used cautiously, as Zoledronic acid is cleared renally and nephrotoxicity is a known risk at higher doses. Calcium-supporting herbs such as Shankh Bhasma (used as a mineral preparation), Ashwagandha, and Bala may modulate calcium metabolism and bone strength and should be carefully balanced to avoid interfering with the drug's effects. While antioxidant and tissue-repairing herbs like Amalaki and Guduchi are generally safe, their influence on systemic metabolism or immune modulation should be monitored.

Because Zoledronic acid affects bone remodeling and renal function, combining it with herbs that influence mineral balance, kidney function, or systemic inflammation should be done with professional oversight to avoid complications.

Zopiclone (*Imovane, Zimovane*), a non-benzodiazepine sedative-hypnotic used for the short-term treatment of insomnia, acts on GABA receptors to promote sleep and muscle relaxation.

It may interact with various Western and Ayurvedic herbs that influence central nervous system activity, particularly those with sedative, anxiolytic, or cognitive effects.

Among Western herbs, Valerian, Kava, Hops, Skullcap, Passionflower, and Chamomile can intensify the sedative properties of Zopiclone, potentially leading to excessive drowsiness, dizziness, slowed reaction time, or next-day grogginess. St. John's Wort may reduce the effectiveness of Zopiclone by inducing liver enzymes that speed up its clearance, but its serotonergic effects also raise the risk of mood instability or paradoxical reactions when combined with sedatives.

In the Ayurvedic tradition, calming and nervine herbs such as Ashwagandha, Tagara, Jatamansi, and Shankhpushpi may enhance Zopiclone's central nervous system depressant effects, especially in individuals sensitive to sedation. Brahmi and Vacha, which promote cognitive clarity and balance mental function, may interact in more subtle ways with Zopiclone's influence on sleep architecture and mental alertness. While these herbs are often used safely on their own, combining them with Zopiclone can lead to potentiation of effects such as excessive sedation or impaired coordination.

Because Zopiclone affects GABAergic transmission and has a narrow margin for safe sedative use, it should not be taken with herbs that similarly affect sleep, relaxation, or cognition without guidance from a qualified healthcare provider.

Chapter 5:
INTEGRATING PHARMACEUTICAL REMEDIES INTO ALTERNATIVE HEALTH PRACTICES

Collaborating with Medical Professionals
Collaborating with medical professionals is an essential aspect of providing comprehensive care for patients as an alternative health practitioner. By working together with doctors, pharmacists, and other healthcare professionals, you can ensure that your patients receive the best possible treatment plan that integrates both pharmaceutical remedies and alternative therapies.

One key benefit of collaborating with medical professionals is the ability to access their expertise and knowledge in the field of pharmaceutical drugs. Doctors and pharmacists have extensive training and experience in understanding the mechanisms of action, potential side effects, and appropriate dosages of various medications. By consulting with them, you can gain valuable insights into which pharmaceutical remedies may be most effective for your patients' specific health conditions.

In addition, collaborating with medical professionals can help you navigate the complex world of drug interactions. Mixing pharmaceutical drugs with certain herbs, supplements, or alternative therapies can sometimes lead to adverse reactions or diminished effectiveness. By consulting with doctors and pharmacists, you can ensure that your treatment plan is safe and optimized for your patients' well-being.

Moreover, building strong relationships with medical professionals can also enhance your credibility as an alternative health practitioner. When doctors and pharmacists see that you are committed to working collaboratively and prioritizing your patients' health and safety, they are more likely to refer patients to you for complementary care. This can help you expand your practice and reach a wider audience of individuals seeking holistic healthcare options.

Overall, collaborating with medical professionals is a win-win situation for both you as an alternative health practitioner and for your patients. By combining your expertise in alternative therapies with the knowledge and skills of doctors and pharmacists, you can provide a more comprehensive and effective treatment approach that addresses the whole person's health needs. Remember, teamwork makes the dream work when it comes to delivering high-quality care in the realm of pharmaceutical drugs and drug therapy for alternative health practitioners.

Monitoring and Evaluating Drug Therapy

Monitoring and evaluating drug therapy is a crucial aspect of providing effective treatment for patients. As alternative health practitioners, it is essential to understand the importance of regularly assessing the effectiveness and safety of pharmaceutical remedies in order to optimize patient outcomes. By closely monitoring the progress of patients and evaluating their response to drug therapy, practitioners can make necessary adjustments to the treatment plan and ensure that patients are receiving the most appropriate care.

One key aspect of monitoring drug therapy is keeping detailed records of each patient's treatment journey. This includes documenting the medications prescribed, dosages, frequency of administration, and any side effects or adverse reactions that may occur. By maintaining thorough and accurate records, practitioners can track the progress of patients over time and identify any patterns or trends that may indicate the need for changes to the treatment plan.

In addition to tracking medication use, practitioners should also regularly assess patients' symptoms and overall health status. This may involve conducting physical exams, ordering laboratory tests, or using other diagnostic tools to monitor the impact of drug therapy on the patient's condition. By closely monitoring patients' progress, practitioners can ensure that medications are working as intended and make informed decisions about any necessary adjustments to the treatment plan.

Evaluating drug therapy involves assessing both the benefits and potential risks of pharmaceutical remedies. Practitioners should be vigilant in monitoring for any signs of drug interactions, adverse effects, or other complications that may arise during treatment. By staying informed about the latest research and guidelines for drug therapy, practitioners can make evidence-based decisions to optimize patient outcomes and minimize the risk of harm.

In conclusion, monitoring and evaluating drug therapy is a critical component of providing safe and effective care to patients as alternative health practitioners. By keeping detailed records, regularly assessing patients' progress, and evaluating the benefits and risks of pharmaceutical remedies, practitioners can ensure that patients receive the most appropriate and personalized treatment. By staying informed and proactive in monitoring drug therapy, practitioners can help their patients achieve optimal health outcomes and improve their overall quality of life.

Chapter 6:
HERBAL AND NUTRITIONAL SUPPLEMENTS AS COMPLEMENTARY TREATMENTS

Understanding Herbal Remedies

Herbal remedies have been used for centuries as a natural alternative to pharmaceutical drugs. Alternative health practitioners often turn to herbs as a way to treat a variety of ailments and promote overall wellness in their patients. Understanding the benefits and potential risks of herbal remedies is essential for any practitioner looking to incorporate them into their practice.

One of the key advantages of herbal remedies is their natural origins. Unlike pharmaceutical drugs, which are often synthesized in a laboratory, herbal remedies come from plants and other natural sources. This can make them more appealing to patients who prefer a more holistic approach to their healthcare. Additionally, many herbs have been used for generations in traditional medicine systems around the world, providing a wealth of knowledge on their potential benefits and uses.

However, it is important to note that not all herbal remedies are safe or effective. Just because a remedy is natural does not mean it is free from potential side effects or interactions with other medications. Alternative health practitioners must thoroughly research each herb they recommend to ensure its safety and efficacy for their patients. Consulting with a qualified herbalist or pharmacist can also provide valuable insights into the best practices for incorporating herbal remedies into a treatment plan.

Another important consideration when using herbal remedies is the quality of the product. Not all herbal supplements are created equal, and some may contain contaminants or adulterants that can be harmful to patients. Alternative health practitioners should only recommend products from reputable manufacturers that adhere to strict quality control standards.

Additionally, practitioners should educate their patients on how to properly dose and use herbal remedies to maximize their effectiveness and minimize the risk of adverse effects.

Herbal remedies can be a valuable addition to an alternative health practitioner's toolkit when used responsibly and with caution. By understanding the benefits and potential risks of herbal remedies, practitioners can provide their patients with safe and effective treatment options that align with their holistic approach to healthcare. With proper research, quality control, and patient education, herbal remedies can play a significant role in promoting overall wellness and improving health outcomes for patients.

Incorporating Nutritional Supplements

Incorporating nutritional supplements into drug therapy can be a powerful tool for alternative health practitioners looking to optimize their patients' health and well-being. Nutritional supplements can complement pharmaceutical drugs by providing essential vitamins, minerals, and nutrients that may be lacking in the patient's diet. This subchapter will explore the benefits of incorporating nutritional supplements into drug therapy and provide guidelines for how to do so effectively.

One of the key benefits of incorporating nutritional supplements into drug therapy is the ability to address nutrient deficiencies that may be contributing to the patient's health issues. Many pharmaceutical drugs can deplete essential nutrients from the body, leading to a range of health problems. By supplementing with vitamins and minerals, alternative health practitioners can help to restore balance and improve the overall effectiveness of drug therapy.

In addition to addressing nutrient deficiencies, nutritional supplements can also support the body's natural healing processes and promote overall health and well-being. For example, antioxidants such as vitamin C and E can help to protect the body from oxidative stress and reduce inflammation, while omega-3 fatty acids can support heart health and cognitive function. By incorporating these supplements into drug therapy, alternative health practitioners can help their patients achieve better outcomes and improve their quality of life.

When incorporating nutritional supplements into drug therapy, it is important for alternative health practitioners to consider the potential interactions between supplements and pharmaceutical drugs. Some supplements may enhance the effects of certain drugs, while others may interfere with their absorption or metabolism. It is important to consult with a healthcare provider or pharmacist to ensure that the supplements being used are safe and effective for the patient's specific needs.

In conclusion, incorporating nutritional supplements into drug therapy can be a valuable tool for alternative health practitioners looking to enhance the effectiveness of pharmaceutical remedies. By addressing nutrient deficiencies, supporting the body's natural healing processes, and promoting overall health and well-being, supplements can help to optimize patient outcomes and improve quality of life. With careful consideration of potential interactions and guidance from healthcare providers, alternative health practitioners can successfully integrate nutritional supplements into their treatment plans to achieve the best possible results for their patients.

Combining Pharmaceutical Drugs with Natural Remedies

Combining pharmaceutical drugs with natural remedies can be a powerful approach to treating various health conditions. As alternative health practitioners, it is important to understand how these two modalities can work together to provide optimal care for your patients. By integrating pharmaceutical drugs with natural remedies, you can create a comprehensive treatment plan that addresses the root cause of the problem while also supporting the body's natural healing mechanisms.

When combining pharmaceutical drugs with natural remedies, it is crucial to consider potential interactions between the two. Some natural remedies may enhance or inhibit the effects of certain medications, leading to adverse reactions or decreased efficacy. It is essential to thoroughly research and understand how each medication and natural remedy works in the body to ensure they can be safely used together. Consulting with a healthcare provider or pharmacist who is knowledgeable about drug interactions can help guide you in creating a safe and effective treatment plan. Potential interactions between herbs and pharmaceutical drugs are detailed in chapter four of this work.

One benefit of combining pharmaceutical drugs with natural remedies is the potential for reduced side effects. Natural remedies such as herbs, supplements, and lifestyle modifications can help support the body's systems and reduce the need for higher doses of medications. This can lead to a more gentle and holistic approach to treatment, promoting overall wellness and reducing the risk of adverse reactions. By using a combination of pharmaceutical drugs and natural remedies, you can tailor treatment plans to meet the individual needs of each patient, taking into account their unique health concerns and preferences.

Incorporating natural remedies into a treatment plan can also help address underlying imbalances or deficiencies that may be contributing to a patient's symptoms. Pharmaceutical drugs are often used to manage symptoms, but they may not always address the root cause of the issue. By combining pharmaceutical drugs with natural remedies that target specific imbalances or deficiencies, you can create a more comprehensive approach to healing that promotes long-term health and well-being. This integrative approach can help patients achieve optimal results and improve their overall quality of life.

As alternative health practitioners, it is important to stay informed about the latest research and developments in the field of drug therapy. By understanding how pharmaceutical drugs and natural remedies can work together, you can offer your patients a more holistic and personalized approach to treatment. By combining the best of both worlds, you can create innovative and effective treatment plans that support the body's innate healing abilities and promote optimal health and wellness for your patients.

Practical Tips for Integrating Drug Therapy in Alternative Health Practices

As alternative health practitioners, incorporating drug therapy into your practice can be a daunting task. However, with the right knowledge and guidance, you can effectively integrate pharmaceutical remedies into your alternative health practices. In this subchapter, we will provide you with practical tips to help you navigate the world of drug therapy and ensure the safety and well-being of your clients.

First and foremost, it is essential to stay informed about the latest developments in pharmaceutical drugs and drug therapy. This includes staying up-to-date on new medications, potential side effects, and drug interactions. Attend seminars, workshops, and conferences related to drug therapy to expand your knowledge and stay current with industry trends.

When integrating drug therapy into your practice, always prioritize the safety and well-being of your clients. Conduct a thorough assessment of each client's medical history, current medications, and any allergies or sensitivities they may have. This will help you determine the most appropriate pharmaceutical remedies for their specific needs and reduce the risk of adverse reactions.

Collaboration with other healthcare professionals, such as pharmacists and physicians, is crucial when incorporating drug therapy into your alternative health practices. Consult with these professionals to ensure that your clients receive the best possible care and that any potential drug interactions or contraindications are identified and addressed promptly.

Lastly, always be transparent with your clients about the use of pharmaceutical remedies in your practice. Educate them about the benefits and risks of drug therapy, and involve them in the decision-making process regarding their treatment plan. By fostering open communication and trust with your clients, you can ensure a collaborative and effective approach to integrating drug therapy into your alternative health practices.

Chapter 7: RESOURCES AND FURTHER READING

Recommended Books and Journals

As Alternative Health Practitioners, staying up to date with the latest information on pharmaceutical drugs and drug therapy is crucial to providing effective care for your clients. To help you expand your knowledge and enhance your practice, here are some recommended books and journals that cover a wide range of topics related to pharmaceutical remedies.

One highly recommended book for Alternative Health Practitioners is "*Pharmacology for the Health Care Professions*" by Christine M. Thorp. This comprehensive guide provides a detailed overview of pharmacology principles and their application in healthcare settings. It covers topics such as drug classifications, mechanisms of action, and dosage calculations, making it an essential resource for practitioners looking to deepen their understanding of pharmaceutical drugs.

For practitioners interested in exploring the latest research and developments in drug therapy, the "*Journal of Pharmaceutical Sciences*" is an invaluable resource. This peer-reviewed journal publishes cutting-edge research on drug discovery, development, and delivery, providing practitioners with access to the most current information in the field. Subscribing to this journal can help you stay informed about emerging trends and advancements in pharmaceutical science.

Another recommended book for Alternative Health Practitioners is "*Pharmacotherapy: A Pathophysiologic Approach*" by Joseph T. DiPiro. This comprehensive text offers a detailed examination of the pathophysiology of various diseases and the pharmacologic treatment options available. It covers a wide range of therapeutic areas, including cardiovascular, respiratory, and infectious diseases, making it a valuable resource for practitioners seeking to improve their clinical decision-making skills.

Very useful reference texts include Alan Gaby's *A-Z Guide to Drug-Herb Vitamin Interactions*, *Herb Toxicities and Drug Interactions: A Formula Approach* by Fred Jennes and Bob Flaws, and *Stockley's Herbal Medicines Interactions* edited by Elizabeth Williamson et al., and the *PDR for Herbal Medicines*, edited by T. Fleming et al.

For practitioners looking to explore alternative approaches to drug therapy, the "*Journal of Alternative and Complementary Medicine*" is an excellent resource. This peer-reviewed journal publishes research on complementary and alternative therapies, including herbal remedies, acupuncture, and mind-body practices. Subscribing to this journal can help you broaden your understanding of holistic approaches to healthcare and incorporate them into your practice.

In conclusion, staying informed about pharmaceutical drugs and drug therapy is essential for Alternative Health Practitioners looking to provide the best possible care for their clients. By exploring the recommended books and journals mentioned above, you can deepen your knowledge, expand your skill set, and stay current on the latest advancements in pharmaceutical remedies. Whether you are interested in traditional pharmacology or alternative approaches to drug therapy, these resources can help you enhance your practice and improve patient outcomes.

Glossary of Drug Terms

Analgesic – Relieves pain without causing loss of consciousness.
Examples: Acetaminophen (Tylenol), Ibuprofen (Advil), Naproxen (Aleve).
Anesthetic – Induces loss of sensation or consciousness, either locally or generally.
Examples: Lidocaine (local), Propofol (general).
Antacid – Neutralizes stomach acid to relieve heartburn and indigestion.
Examples: Calcium carbonate (Tums), Magnesium hydroxide (Milk of Magnesia).
Antibiotic – Kills or inhibits the growth of bacteria, treating bacterial infections.
Examples: Amoxicillin, Azithromycin, Ciprofloxacin.
Anticoagulant – Reduces blood clotting, helping to prevent strokes and heart attacks.
Examples: Warfarin (Coumadin), Heparin, Apixaban (Eliquis).
Anticonvulsant – Prevents or reduces the frequency and severity of seizures.
Examples: Phenytoin (Dilantin), Valproic acid (Depakote), Lamotrigine.
Antidepressant – Treats depression, anxiety, and other mood disorders.
Examples: Fluoxetine (Prozac), Sertraline (Zoloft), Venlafaxine (Effexor).
Antidiabetic – Controls blood sugar levels in people with diabetes.
Examples: Glipizide (Glucotrol – stimulates insulin release), Metformin (Glucophage – reduces glucose production in the liver and improves insulin sensitivity).

Antidiarrheal – Slows down bowel movements and reduces diarrhea.
Examples: Loperamide (Imodium), Bismuth subsalicylate (Pepto-Bismol).
Antiemetic – Prevents or reduces nausea and vomiting.
Examples: Ondansetron (Zofran), Metoclopramide (Reglan).
Antifungal – Treats fungal infections of the skin, nails, or internal organs.
Examples: Fluconazole (Diflucan), Clotrimazole (Lotrimin).
Antihistamine – Blocks histamine receptors to treat allergies, hives, and sometimes motion sickness.
Examples: Diphenhydramine (Benadryl), Loratadine (Claritin), Cetirizine (Zyrtec).
Antihypertensive – Lowers high blood pressure to reduce the risk of stroke and heart disease.
Examples: Lisinopril (ACE inhibitor), Amlodipine (calcium channel blocker), Losartan (ARB).
Anti-inflammatory – Reduces inflammation, pain, and swelling.
Examples: NSAIDs like Ibuprofen, Corticosteroids like Prednisone.
Antipsychotic – Manages symptoms of psychotic disorders like schizophrenia and bipolar disorder.
Examples: Risperidone (Risperdal), Olanzapine (Zyprexa), Aripiprazole (Abilify).
Antiviral – Inhibits the replication of viruses and can be used to treat infections like herpes and influenza.
Examples: Acyclovir (Zovirax), Oseltamivir (Tamiflu).
Anxiolytic – Reduces anxiety and may induce relaxation.
Examples: Lorazepam (Ativan), Diazepam (Valium).
Beta-blocker – Slows heart rate, lowers blood pressure, and decreases heart workload.

Examples: Metoprolol (Lopressor), Atenolol (Tenormin), Propranolol (Inderal).
Biologic – A drug derived from living cells, used to treat diseases like rheumatoid arthritis, psoriasis, and cancer.
Examples: Adalimumab (Humira), Infliximab (Remicade).
Bronchodilator – Opens airways in the lungs, making breathing easier.
Examples: Albuterol (ProAir, Ventolin), Salmeterol (Serevent).
Calcium Channel Blocker – Relaxes and widens blood vessels by inhibiting calcium movement into the heart and artery cells.
Examples: Diltiazem (Cardizem), Amlodipine (Norvasc).
Chemotherapeutic Agent – Targets and kills rapidly dividing cells, primarily used in cancer treatment.
Examples: Doxorubicin, Paclitaxel.
Corticosteroid – Synthetic hormones that reduce inflammation and suppress the immune system.
Examples: Prednisone, Hydrocortisone, Dexamethasone.
Cytotoxic Agent – Destroys or damages cells, often used in cancer therapies.
Examples: Cyclophosphamide, Cisplatin.
Diuretic – Increases urine production to help remove excess fluid from the body, often used in hypertension and heart failure.
Examples: Furosemide (Lasix), Hydrochlorothiazide (HCTZ), Spironolactone.
Expectorant – Helps thin mucus so it can be coughed out more easily.
Examples: Guaifenesin (Mucinex).
Hallucinogen – Causes altered perceptions, thoughts, and feelings.
Examples: Lysergic acid diethylamide (LSD), Psilocybin (magic mushrooms).

Hormone Replacement Therapy (HRT) – Supplements declining hormone levels due to menopause, aging, or disease.
Examples: Estradiol, Testosterone.
Hypnotic – Induces and maintains sleep.
Examples: Zolpidem (Ambien), Eszopiclone (Lunesta).
Immunosuppressant – Suppresses the immune system to prevent transplant rejection or treat autoimmune diseases.
Examples: Cyclosporine, Methotrexate, Tacrolimus.
Insulin – A hormone replacement therapy for type 1 and advanced type 2 diabetes, regulating blood sugar levels.
Types: Rapid-acting (lispro), Long-acting (glargine).
Laxative – Promotes bowel movements to relieve constipation.
Examples: Senna (Senokot), Polyethylene glycol (MiraLAX), Psyllium (Metamucil).
Local Anesthetic – Blocks nerve signals in a specific area of the body.
Examples: Lidocaine, Bupivacaine.
Mood Stabilizer – Helps control extreme mood swings, particularly in bipolar disorder.
Examples: Lithium, Lamotrigine (Lamictal), Valproate.
Muscle Relaxant – Relieves muscle spasms and stiffness.
Examples: Cyclobenzaprine (Flexeril), Baclofen.
Narcotic (Opioid) – Powerful painkillers that can cause dependence and respiratory depression.
Examples: Morphine, Oxycodone, Hydrocodone.
Neuroleptic – Older term for antipsychotic medications; mainly treats psychosis.
Opioid – Binds to opioid receptors to block pain signals in the brain and body.
Examples: Fentanyl, Codeine, Buprenorphine.

Oral Hypoglycemic Agent – Reduces blood glucose levels orally in type 2 diabetes.
Examples: Glipizide (stimulates pancreas to release insulin), Metformin (reduces liver glucose production).
Probiotic – Live microorganisms that promote a healthy digestive tract and immune system.
Examples: Lactobacillus, Bifidobacterium.
Proton Pump Inhibitor (PPI) – Blocks the enzyme responsible for acid production in the stomach, used to treat GERD.
Examples: Omeprazole (Prilosec), Pantoprazole (Protonix).
Sedative – Induces relaxation, calmness, and often drowsiness.
Examples: Diazepam (Valium), Lorazepam (Ativan).
Stimulant – Increases alertness, attention, and energy by raising the levels of key chemicals in the brain.
Examples: Caffeine, Amphetamine salts (Adderall), Methylphenidate (Ritalin).
Statin – Lowers cholesterol levels to reduce the risk of cardiovascular disease.
Examples: Atorvastatin (Lipitor), Rosuvastatin (Crestor).
Steroid – Includes both corticosteroids (anti-inflammatory) and anabolic steroids (muscle growth).
Corticosteroid examples: Prednisone; Anabolic examples: Testosterone derivatives.
Thrombolytic – Breaks apart dangerous clots in blood vessels.
Examples: Alteplase (tPA), Streptokinase.
Tranquilizer – A general term for drugs that calm or sedate; includes both major tranquilizers (antipsychotics) and minor tranquilizers (anxiolytics).
Examples: Diazepam (minor), Haloperidol (major).

Vaccine – Stimulates the immune system to prevent infectious diseases.
Examples: Influenza vaccine, COVID-19 vaccines (mRNA, adenovirus vector types).

Bibliography

DiPiro, Joseph T. et al. *Pharmacotherapy: A Pathophysiologic Approach* (9th ed.), McGraw-Hill Medical (New York NY USA) 2014 ISBN 978-0-07-180053-2

Fleming, Thomas et al., *PDR for Herbal Medicines,* Medical Economics Co., Inc. (Montvale, NJ USA) 2000 ISBN 1-56363-361-2

Gaby Alan R., ed., *A-Z Guide to Drug-Herb-Vitamin Interactions*, Three Rivers Press (New York NY USA) 2006 ISBN 978-0-307-33664-4

Jennes, Fred & Flaws, B., *Herb Toxicities and Drug Interactions: A Formula Approach*, Blue Poppy Press (Boulder, CO USA) 2004 ISBN 1-891845-26-8

Thorp, Christine M., *Pharmacology for the Health Care Professions,* Wiley-Blackwell (Oxford UK) 2008 ISBN 978-0-470-51-18-6

Williamson, Elizabeth, et al., *Stockley's Herbal Medicines Interactions*, Pharmaceutical Press (London UK) 2009 ISBN 978 0 85369 760 2

www.ingramcontent.com/pod-product-compliance
Lightning Source LLC
Chambersburg PA
CBHW052243220526
45471CB00001B/162